A Nurse's Guide to Caring for Cancer Survivors: Lung Cancer

Wendye DiSalvo, DNP, APRN-BC, AOCN®
Nurse Practitioner
Norris Cotton Cancer Center
Dartmouth-Hitchcock Medical Center
Lebanon, New Hampshire

Series Editor
Lisa Kennedy Sheldon, PhD, APRN-BC, AOCNP®
Oncology Nurse Practitioner, St. Joseph Hospital
Nashua, New Hampshire
Assistant Professor, University of Massachusetts–Boston
Boston, Massachusetts

JONES AND BARTLETT PUBLISHERS
Sudbury, Massachusetts
BOSTON   TORONTO   LONDON   SINGAPORE

World Headquarters

Jones and Bartlett Publishers
40 Tall Pine Drive
Sudbury, MA 01776
978-443-5000
info@jbpub.com
www.jbpub.com

Jones and Bartlett Publishers
Canada
6339 Ormindale Way
Mississauga, Ontario L5V 1J2
Canada

Jones and Bartlett Publishers
International
Barb House, Barb Mews
London W6 7PA
United Kingdom

Jones and Bartlett's books and products are available through most bookstores and online booksellers. To contact Jones and Bartlett Publishers directly, call 800-832-0034, fax 978-443-8000, or visit our website, www.jbpub.com.

Substantial discounts on bulk quantities of Jones and Bartlett's publications are available to corporations, professional associations, and other qualified organizations. For details and specific discount information, contact the special sales department at Jones and Bartlett via the above contact information or send an email to specialsales@jbpub.com.

The authors, editors, and publisher have made every effort to provide accurate information. However, they are not responsible for errors, omissions, or for any outcomes related to the use of the contents of this book and take no responsibility for the use of the products and procedures described. Treatments and side effects described in this book may not be applicable to all people; likewise, some people may require a dose or experience a side effect that is not described herein. Drugs and medical devices are discussed that may have limited availability controlled by the Food and Drug Administration (FDA) for use only in a research study or clinical trial. Research, clinical practice, and government regulations often change the accepted standard in this field. When consideration is being given to use of any drug in the clinical setting, the health care provider or reader is responsible for determining FDA status of the drug, reading the package insert, and reviewing prescribing information for the most up-to-date recommendations on dose, precautions, and contraindications, and determining the appropriate usage for the product. This is especially important in the case of drugs that are new or seldom used.

Production Credits
Publisher: Kevin Sullivan
Acquisitions Editor: Emily Ekle
Acquisitions Editor: Amy Sibley
Associate Editor: Patricia Donnelly
Editorial Assistant: Rachel Shuster
Production Editor: Amanda Clerkin
Senior Marketing Manager: Barb Bartoszek
V.P., Manufacturing and Inventory Control: Therese Connell
Composition: DSCS/Absolute Service, Inc.
Cover Designer: Scott Moden
Cover Image: © Iakov Kalinin/ShutterStock, Inc.
Printing and Binding: Cenveo
Cover Printing: Cenveo

Library of Congress Cataloging-in-Publication Data
DiSalvo, Wendye.
    A nurse's guide to caring for cancer survivors: Lung cancer / Wendye DiSalvo.
       p. ; cm.
    Includes bibliographical references and index.
    ISBN-13: 978-0-7637-7260-4 (alk. paper)
    ISBN-10: 0-7637-7260-7 (alk. paper)
1. Lungs—Cancer—Nursing. I. Title. II. Title: Lung cancer.
    [DNLM: 1. Lung Neoplasms—nursing. 2. Lung Neoplasms—therapy.
3. Nurse-Patient Relations. 4. Survivors. WY 156 K35nb 2010]
    RC280.L8K46 2010
    616.99'424—dc22
                                                                        2009018667
6048

Printed in the United States of America
13 12 11 10 09   10 9 8 7 6 5 4 3 2 1

Table of Contents

Contributing Authors

Wendy E. Bayles-Dazet, APRN-BC
Nurse Practitioner
Department of Psychiatry
Dartmouth-Hitchcock Medical Center
Lebanon, NH

Charlotte Bell, MSW
Oncology Social Worker
St. Joseph Hospital
Nashua, NH

Kasia Bloch, MS, CGC
Certified Genetic Counselor
Norris Cotton Cancer Center
Dartmouth-Hitchcock Medical Center
Lebanon, NH

Jeannine M. Brant, PhD, APRN-CNS, AOCN®
Oncology Clinical Nurse Specialist/
Nurse Scientist
Billings Clinic Cancer Care
Billings, MT

Paula A. Caron, MS, APRN-BC, AOCN®
Nurse Practitioner
Norris Cotton Cancer Center
Dartmouth-Hitchcock Medical Center
Lebanon, NH

Wendye DiSalvo, DNP, APRN-BC, AOCN®
Nurse Practitioner
Norris Cotton Cancer Center
Dartmouth-Hitchcock Medical Center
Lebanon, NH

Charlene Gates, PT
Physical Therapist
Norris Cotton Cancer Center
Dartmouth-Hitchcock Medical Center
Lebanon, NH

Stephanie Marcotte, RN, BA, BSN, OCN®
Bryan, TX

Jeannine Mills, MS, RD, LD
Registered Dietician
Norris Cotton Cancer Center
Dartmouth-Hitchcock Medical Center
Lebanon, NH

Claire Pace, RN, OCN®
Nurse Practitioner
Norris Cotton Cancer Center
Dartmouth-Hitchcock Medical Center
Lebanon, NH

Lisa Kennedy Sheldon, PhD, APRN-BC, AOCNP®
Assistant Professor
University of Massachusetts–Boston
Boston, MA
Oncology Nurse Practitioner
St. Joseph Hospital
Nashua, NH

Karen A. Skalla, MSN, APRN-BC, AOCN®
Nurse Practitioner
Norris Cotton Cancer Center
Dartmouth-Hitchcock Medical Center
Lebanon, NH

Ellen M. Lavoie Smith, PhD, APRN-BC, AOCNP®
Assistant Professor
University of Michigan School of Nursing
Ann Arbor, MI

Laura Urquhart, MS, APRN-BC, OCN®
Nurse Practitioner
Norris Cotton Cancer Center
Dartmouth-Hitchcock Medical Center
Lebanon, NH

Jennifer Welch, RN, BSN, OCN®
Oncology Nurse
Beth Israel Hospital
Boston, MA

About the Editor

Lisa Kennedy Sheldon, PhD, APRN-BC, AOCNP®, is an assistant professor at the University of Massachusetts–Boston and an oncology nurse practitioner at St. Joseph Hospital in Nashua, New Hampshire. A graduate of Saint Anselm College and Boston College, Dr. Sheldon received her Doctor of Philosophy from the College of Nursing at the University of Utah with a focus on cancer control and research. Her program of research focuses on patient–provider communication, patient distress, and oncology nursing. Dr. Sheldon has written extensively on nursing issues with recent publications including *Communication for Nurses: Talking with Patients, Second Edition*; *Quick Look Nursing: Oxygenation*; and numerous articles. Dr. Sheldon also serves as an associate editor for the *Clinical Journal of Oncology Nursing*. In addition to teaching, Dr. Sheldon provides direct care to oncology patients receiving treatment as well as presents locally and nationally on communication research, nursing care delivery, and oncology issues. She is a founding partner of Barrett & Sheldon LLC, a corporation focusing on healthcare research and nursing services development.

About the Author

Wendye DiSalvo, DNP, APRN-BC, AOCN®, is a thoracic oncology nurse practitioner at Dartmouth Hitchcock Medical Center in Lebanon, New Hampshire. A graduate of the University of Maryland Nursing School, Mrs. DiSalvo received her Master of Nursing degree from Syracuse University. She is currently enrolled in the Doctor of Nursing Practice program at MGH Institute of Health Professions in Boston, Massachusetts, and will graduate this December. Mrs. DiSalvo has published a chapter on lung cancer in *Primary Care*. She was the leader of the Dyspnea Putting Evidence into Practice (PEP) card team for the Oncology Nursing Society and the lead author of Putting Evidence into Practice Interventions for Dyspnea. Mrs. DiSalvo speaks locally and nationally on symptom management and the treatment of lung cancer. In addition to providing care to thoracic oncology patients, she also provides tobacco treatment interventions in the survivorship clinic run by nurse practitioners.

CHAPTER ONE

Introduction to Survivorship

I n the last three decades, tremendous breakthroughs in cancer research have led to changes in clinical practice, improving survival for people with cancer. When the National Cancer Act was signed into law in 1971, the refrain was, "Make cancer a national crusade." At that time, the primary focus was on treatment aimed at curing the disease. Now, it is estimated that 62% of adults diagnosed with cancer today can expect to be alive in 5 years, and 75% of pediatric cancer survivors will be alive after 10 years. Although many people are cured of their cancer, some will be living with their disease as a chronic condition. Others will be coping with the long-term side effects of their treatment. All will be changed by their experience with a diagnosis of cancer.

The concept of *cancer survivorship* was introduced in the field of oncology in 1986 by the National Coalition for Cancer Survivorship (NCCS). Because of the improvements in prevention, detection, and treatment of cancer, there is a growing group of people who have been diagnosed with this disease, and more than 12 million cancer survivors in the United States. Cancer survivors have been defined in different ways, from those people who have just been diagnosed to those having finished treatment. However, cancer also affects another group of people: families and caregivers. Three out of four families in the United States have at least one family member diagnosed with cancer. To acknowledge the broader effects of cancer, the National Cancer Institute (NCI) has included another group in the definition of cancer survivor, *secondary survivors*, which includes the caregivers and family members of cancer survivors. This broader definition creates awareness of the impact of a cancer diagnosis on the family members and a greater voice for caregivers in policies and legislation. This group has increasingly inspired legislation, including the Family and Medical Leave Act (FMLA) of 1993.

For the purposes of this manual, the definition of a cancer survivor is:

> *Anyone diagnosed with cancer, from the time of diagnosis through the rest of his or her life, including the end of life, and the family members and caregivers of the cancer survivor.*

The 2004 Institute of Medicine (IOM) report, *From Cancer Patient to Cancer Survivor: Lost in Transition*, provided detailed recommendations directed toward cancer patients and their advocates, including healthcare providers, leaders in academics and policy making, insurers, employers, researchers, and the public and their elected representatives. One group, the healthcare providers, often struggle with how to coordinate the needs of cancer survivors because of the complexity of cancer care and its long-term effects. The healthcare system requires changes to address the unique needs of cancer survivors and coordinate care among the providers.

Primary treatment for cancer is often rigorous and multimodal, requiring the coordination of care among multiple healthcare providers. Some adjuvant therapies, such as hormone blockade, may continue for years after the initial treatment.

The late effects of cancer treatment are often unrecognized and may become apparent years after the initial treatment. Additionally, the risk of a second cancer is significant for certain cancers and their treatments. Because of the risk of recurrence and the potential development of secondary cancers, surveillance and screening tests are necessary for years after the initial treatment. Because of the ongoing possibility of further treatment, the perception of cancer has begun to change. Increasingly, it is viewed as a chronic illness, much like diabetes with remissions and exacerbations requiring additional treatment. Because of its chronic nature, cancer treatment may be necessary during the time of survivorship to prolong survival, relieve symptoms, and improve quality of life.

Oncology nurses are in a unique position to facilitate the care of cancer survivors and support them before, during, and after a diagnosis of cancer. Oncology nurses are not only involved in cancer treatment; they are also educators, navigators, counselors, advanced practice nurses, and advocates for people with cancer. The significance of their role was highlighted in the 2004 IOM report and the upcoming report from the IOM National Cancer Policy Forum on the oncology workforce.

The promotion of healthy behaviors is often neglected in patients receiving treatment for cancer. The focus of follow-up care is often screening and surveillance for cancer, whereas other health issues may need addressing by providers. Because of the higher rates of survival, survivors need to continue or begin healthy behaviors, including good nutrition, regular exercise, and smoking cessation. Often, a diagnosis of cancer is a "wake-up call," and people are motivated to take care of themselves in new ways. Oncology nurses are in an important position to promote healthy behaviors and refer survivors to additional resources.

After the initial diagnosis and treatment, there is currently no smooth transition into cancer survivorship. Follow-up care is often scattered among the oncology specialists and primary care providers, with resulting confusion and inadequate follow up, and the creation of fear in patients. Increasingly, programs for survivorship are being created, using oncology nurses and nurse practitioners to address the needs of cancer survivors. Because cancer may have many different diagnoses, treatments, and long-term survival patterns, this manual has been created for a specific cancer diagnosis to help oncology nurses tailor their care for survivors. Ultimately, it is hoped that this manual will increase awareness of the needs of cancer survivors and improve their outcomes and quality of life before, during, and after cancer treatment.

✺ Addendum

The care of cancer survivors is evolving daily. Recently, new treatment plan and summaries both in a generic format for any cancer and specific formats for breast and colon cancer survivors have been posted on the American Society of Clinical Oncology (ASCO) Web site. Additionally, treatment summaries for survivors with small cell and non-small cell cancer are available on cancer.net. Finally, generic, patient-friendly treatment summaries are currently being developed by the American Cancer Society and will be available shortly on ACS Web site in the new survivorship link.

Web Sites

American Cancer Society (ACS) Web site will post treatment summary in the Fall 2009 on the acs web site: http://www.cancer.org

American Society of Clinical Oncology (ASCO) Web site for breast and lung cancer as well as a generic form for any cancer: http://www.cancer.net/patient/Survivorship/ASCO+Cancer+Treatment+Summaries

Lance Armstrong Foundation (LAF) LIVESTRONG Website: http://www.livestrong.org/atf/cf/%7BFB6FFD43-0E4C-4414-8B37-0D001EFBDC49%7D/medical_summary.pdf

CHAPTER TWO

Overview of Cancer Diagnosis and Treatment Modalities: Lung Cancer

🎗 Introduction

In 1971 the National Cancer Act was signed into law, and the refrain was, "Make cancer a national crusade." In the United States the number of cancer survivors has tripled since 1971. The number of survivors is growing by 2% a year. Because of earlier detection, improved treatment modalities, and supportive care of family and friends, over 10 million people have joined the ranks of cancer survivors (Travis & Yahalom, 2008). Until recently survivorship was defined as being alive 5 years after treatment. The National Cancer Institute (NCI) defines cancer survivor as anyone who has been diagnosed with cancer from the time of diagnosis through the balance of his or her life. The NCI includes family members and loved ones as part of survivorship family (NCI, 2008).

Lung cancer is one of the most common cancers in the world. In 2009 in the United States, the estimated number of new lung cancer diagnoses will be 205,020 individuals, and the estimated deaths from lung cancer, which includes non-small cell and small cell combined, will be 161,840 individuals (NCI, 2008). In the past 30 years the survival has increased from 13% to 16% (American Cancer Society [ACS], 2008).

Utilizing the NCI definition of survivor there are many survivors because of the high incidence of the disease. However, defining a time frame of 5-year or disease-free survival, the number of survivors is significantly reduced to a smaller number of patients, thus limiting research opportunities. Survival for patients with non-small cell lung cancer (NSCLC) is dependent on stage and appropriate treatment strategies. Survival diminishes as the stages progress from stage I to stage IV disease. In small cell lung cancer (SCLC) survival is measured at 2 years, with very few survivors at 5 years (Sarna, Grannis, & Coscarelli, 2008).

At some time over the course of their illness, lung cancer survivors and their families experience uncertainty, which can negatively affect disease outcomes and psychosocial adaptation (McCormick, 2002). The fear of recurrence, morbidity, and long-term side effects may mean that the condition becomes a chronic one for many survivors. Mishel (1990) defined uncertainty in chronic illness as the condition of living with an incapacitating condition in which the person continuously questions the risk of recurrence, progression of disease, and/or his or her unknown future. Therefore, uncertainty in a chronic illness such as lung cancer influences daily activities, negatively influences well-being, and is significantly related to emotional distress (Taylor-Piliate & Molassiotis, 2001).

❀ Background

In the United States and worldwide, lung cancer is a health threat of enormous proportions. Although the incidence of lung cancer is declining in the United States, the disease is rising globally and is directly related to the use of tobacco products (World Health Organization [WHO], 2008). As smoking has declined in the United States, the incidence of lung cancer among men has declined. Significant increase in the rates of smoking among women occurred approximately 20 years later than those in men, with an ensuing delay in increased cases of lung cancer that peaked in the 1990s. Recent evidence suggests that the incidence of lung cancer as well as death rates are now declining among women (Jemal *et al.*, 2008). Approximately 85% of lung cancers could be prevented if the use of tobacco products were eliminated. Thus, primary prevention is needed in order to reduce the incidence of lung cancer (Davies, Houlihan, & Joyce, 2004). The WHO estimates that there are 1.3 billion smokers globally, with an estimated tobacco-related mortality of 10 million deaths by 2030. In the United States, there are 45 million adult cigarette smokers, with 435,000 tobacco-related deaths annually. The sequelae of tobacco use accounts for serious illness in 8.6 million Americans per year. Because of this significant morbidity and mortality, treatment of tobacco addiction is paramount (WHO, 2008). In addition, nearly one third of all lung cancers are caused by smoking. Despite this statistic, it has been estimated that 20% of cancer survivors continue to smoke because of the fatalistic belief that it is too late to quit. On the contrary, cessation of tobacco use has been associated with improved tolerance to treatment, improved survival, and a decreased risk of developing a secondary cancer (Gritz, 2006). (See Chapter 6 for evidence-based interventions.)

Lung cancer also occurs in people who have never smoked. Environmental tobacco smoke (ETS) or second-hand smoke, domestic air pollution, work-related risk factors, radon exposure, and genetics are also implicated in the development of lung cancer (Houlihan, 2004).

The international standard for the histological classification of lung tumors, as delineated by the WHO and the International Association for the Study of Lung Cancer (IASLC), is NSCLC and SCLC. Tumors are made up of sheets of epithelial cells, which range from poorly to well differentiated in classification. Forty percent of all lung cancers are adenocarcinoma in the United States. Non-small cell lung cancer comprises 85% of all lung cancers and includes four histological subtypes: adenocarcinoma, squamous cell carcinoma, adenocarcinoma with bronchioalveolar features, and large cell carcinoma. Small cell lung cancer comprises 15% of all lung cancers, and has a neuroendocrine histology. Because of a change in tobacco smoking habits (filters, light tobacco cigarettes, and degree of inhalation), adenocarcinoma has surpassed squamous and SCLC in incidence (Brambilla, Travis, Colby, Corrin, & Shimosato, 2001).

Non-Small Cell Lung Cancer

In order to have a common language worldwide, lung cancer is staged according to the International Staging System. This system was last revised in 1996 by the American Joint Committee on Cancer (AJCC). The staging is based on primary tumor (T), presence or absence of regional lymph nodes (N), and presence or absence of distant metastasis (M). The stages for NSCLC are: IA, IB, IIA, IIB, IIIA, IIIB, IV (Mountain, 1997). The 5-year survival rates for the stages of disease are 1A (61%), IB (38%), IIA (37%), IIB (21–26%), IIIA (9–13%), IIIB (3–5%), and IV (<1%) (Mountain, 2000). The clinical diagnostic stage of lung cancer is based on tissue sampling, medical history, physical examination, laboratory test, computed tomography (CT), and positron emission tomography (PET) (Greene *et al.*, 2002).

Prognostic Factors

The most important prognostic factor for lung cancer survival is the clinical stage at diagnosis. Cure is directly related to size and location of the tumor at diagnosis. In patients with NSCLC, factors related to longer survival include early stage of disease, good performance status (PS), no significant weight loss, and female gender. Other factors negatively related to survival include male gender, age 60 years or more, presence of the immunohistological factors that include mutation of the tumor suppression gene (p53), and activation of K-ras oncogenes factors (National Comprehensive Cancer Network [NCCN], 2009).

⊗ Treatment

For patients with stage I or II cancer, the best option for cure is surgical intervention, although only 30% of patients are suitable candidates for this (Carney & Hansen, 2000). Radiation and chemotherapy are other modalities employed in the treatment of NSCLC. Chemotherapy is employed after surgery for early stage NSCLC (IB–IIB) as adjuvant therapy and increases the chance of survival (Pignon *et al.*, 2008). See Table 2-1 for a list of chemotherapeutic agents. In patients with stage III disease who are not surgical candidates, a combination of radiation therapy and chemotherapy are used either concurrently or sequentially. See Table 2-2 for a list of chemotherapeutic agents. In stage IV disease, the aim of chemotherapy is to palliate the disease (NCCN, 2009); see Table 2-3 for the listing of chemotherapeutic agents.

TABLE 2-1   Chemotherapeutic Agents Used in Stage I and II Cancer

Chemotherapy agents used for adjuvant therapy after surgical resection	*Chemotherapy agents used for adjuvant therapy for patients with comorbidities or unable to tolerate cisplatin*
Cisplatin used in combination with one of the following:	Paclitaxel
Vinorelbine	Carboplatin
Etoposide	
Vinblastine	
Gemcitabine	
Docetaxel	

From: NCCN Practice Guidelines in Oncology, 2009.

TABLE 2-2   Chemotherapeutic Agents Used in Stage III Cancer

Chemotherapy agents used with concurrent radiation	Sequential chemotherapy agents and radiation
Cisplatin	Cisplatin
Etoposide	Vinblastine
Vinblastine	Paclitaxel
Paclitaxel	Carboplatin
Carboplatin	
Docetaxel	

From: NCCN Practice Guidelines in Oncology, 2009.

There are significant sequelae to any of the interventional modalities. Oncology nurses play a crucial role in the identification and management of immediate and long-term side effects associated with the disease and its treatment. Patient outcomes and quality of life (QOL)

TABLE 2-3   Chemotherapeutic Agents Used in Stage IV Cancer

Chemotherapy agents used in the metastatic setting or recurrence	Chemotherapy agents used for advanced or metastatic disease		
Bevacizumab + chemotherapy	Cisplatin	Vinorelbine	Gemcitabine
	Paclitaxel	Etoposide	
	Docetaxel	Irinotecan	
	Pemetrexed	Ifosfamide	
	Vinblastine	Carboplatin	

From: NCCN Practice Guidelines in Oncology, 2009.

are significantly improved when oncology nurses provide education and support to patients and their families. It is crucial to perform a thorough assessment of patients at each encounter, allowing time for questions and the assimilation of information related to their disease and treatment. Anticipatory guidance as to side effects and potential toxicities is paramount. The most common symptoms associated with lung cancer are cough, hemoptysis, dyspnea, fatigue, chest pain, anorexia, weight loss, depression and anxiety, and insomnia. Nurses play a key role in identifying and managing these symptoms to improve QOL (Houlihan, Inzeo, Joyce, & Tyson, 2004). Please refer to the specific symptom management strategies in Chapter 4.

The side effects related to the administration of chemotherapy include bone marrow suppression, peripheral neuropathy, fatigue, chemotherapy-induced nausea and vomiting (CINV), constipation and/or diarrhea, alopecia, and nail and skin changes. Sequelae to surgical intervention include pain, neuropathy, and dyspnea (Sarna, Grannis, & Coscarelli, 2008). Side effects related to radiation therapy to the thorax include pneumonitis, pharyngitis, esophagitis, skin changes, and dyspnea (Houlihan, Inzeo, Joyce, & Tyson, 2004).

Targeted Therapies

Specific targeted therapies have been developed for the treatment of advanced NSCLC. The recombinant monoclonal antibody bevacizumab (Avastin®) blocks vascular endothelial growth factor (VEGF) and was approved by the US Food and Drug Administration (FDA) in 2007. The antibody is approved for unresectable, locally advanced recurrent or metastatic nonsquamous NSCLC and is used in combination with chemotherapy. This treatment is contraindicated in patients with a history of hemoptysis, untreated central nervous system metastasis, and recent surgery (less than 28 days). Major side effects include hypertension, risk of bleeding, gastrointestinal perforation, protein-uria, and delayed wound healing (NCCN, 2009).

Erlotinib is a small molecule tyrosine kinase inhibitor (TKI) that restrains activity of the epidermal growth factor receptor. It was FDA approved in 2004. It is used in survivors with locally advanced NSCLC who have failed one or more prior chemotherapy regimes. The most common side effects are rash, diarrhea, paronychia, hypertrichosis, and, rarely, interstitial lung disease. Many more targeted therapies are emerging in the treatment of NSCLC.

Other potential complications that nurses should be aware of include paraneoplastic syndromes and oncological emergencies. The most common of the paraneoplastic syndromes are those arising from the endocrine system: hypercalcemia, ectopic adrenocorticotropic hormone syndrome (ACTH), and the syndrome of inappropriate antidiuretic hormone (SIADH) (Tyson, 2004a). Oncological emergencies include superior vena cava syndrome, pericardial effusion, cardiac tamponade, pleural effusion, and malignant spinal cord compression (Tyson, 2004b).

🕸 Small Cell Lung Cancer

Small cell lung cancer is characterized by rapid doubling time, high growth fraction, and propensity to metastasize early. The disease is very responsive to treatment, but relapses quickly and becomes refractory to treatment within 1 to 2 years. It is found almost exclusively in smokers and predominantly in heavy smokers (Ettinger & Aisner, 2006). In 1999, the WHO/IASLC classification of lung and pleural tumors proposed three categories of neuroendocrine lung tumors: classical small cell carcinoma, large cell neuroendocrine cancer, and a combined small cell carcinoma (Junker, Wiethege, & Muller, 2000). Small cell lung cancer is staged as limited or extensive stage. Limited stage is when the cancer is confined to the ipsilateral hemithorax and is contained in a single radiotherapy port. Extensive stage disease is when the cancer is metastatic outside the ipsilateral port. At the time of diagnosis 30% of the patients have limited stage disease and 60–70% have metastatic disease (Joyce, 2004).

Small cell lung cancer is generally more aggressive and metastasizes earlier than NSCLC. A favorable prognosis for SCLC includes limited stage disease, good performance status, female gender, and age less than 70. Survivors with extensive stage disease have a somewhat better prognosis if they have normal levels of the hepatic enzyme lactose dehydrogenase (LDH) and one site of metastatic disease. Poor prognosis is associated with extensive stage disease, weight loss, and extensive tumor bulk (NCCN, 2009).

The staging workup includes tissue diagnosis, physical exam, laboratory values, CT of the chest, liver, adrenals, and head, CT or magnetic resonance imaging (MRI) of the brain, and bone scan. Positron emission tomography scan may be obtained; if used for screening, there is no need for a bone scan (NCCN, 2009). From the time of diagnosis the median survival for limited and extensive stage are 15 and 20 months, respectively. Survival is measured at 2 years with 20 to 40% of limited stage and less than 5% of extensive stage patients being alive. The respective values for 5 years are 10–13% and 1–2%. Adverse prognostic factors are poor PS and weight loss, extensive stage disease, elevated LDH, number of organs affected, male gender, and the presence of paraneoplastic syndrome (Argiris & Murren, 2001). There is a very limited role for surgical resection. Survivors with limited stage disease are treated with systemic chemotherapy and radiation therapy, and those with extensive stage disease receive chemotherapy (Joyce, 2004). Those with limited stage disease after completing definitive combined modality therapy with no evidence of disease progression may benefit from prophylactic cranial irradiation (PCI). Brain metastasis is a frequent finding in SCLC. Prophylactic cranial irradiation helps prevent intracranial relapse and improve survival in survivors who achieved a complete response to induction chemotherapy, those with evidence of significant partial response, and a subset with extensive stage disease with significant tumor response and a good PS. The sequelae to PCI are the potential for neurotoxicity with cognitive decline (Meert *et al.*, 2001). See Table 2-4 for a list of chemotherapeutics utilized in the treatment of SCLC. The nursing considerations are the same as for NSCLC.

TABLE 2-4   Chemotherapeutic Agents Utilized in the Treatment of Small Cell Lung Cancer

Chemotherapy agents for limited stage small cell lung cancer	*Chemotherapy agents for extensive stage small cell lung cancer*	*Subsequent chemotherapies*
Cisplatin or carboplatin combined with etoposide On therapy with chemotherapy and radiotheraphy cisplatin/etoposide is recommended	Cisplatin or Carboplatin Etoposide Cyclophosphamide Doxorubicin Vincristine	*PS 0–2 and relapse <2–3 months* Ifosfamide Paclitaxel Docetaxel Gemcitabine Irinotecan Topotecan *Relapse >2–3 months, the above agents +* Cyclophosphamide Vincristine Doxorubicin Oral etoposide

From: NCCN Practice Guidelines in Oncology, 2009.

❧ Summary

Lung cancer is a significant health threat worldwide. Overall survival is 16% at 5 years. The morbidity and mortality of the disease could be substantially reduced with elimination of tobacco use. Oncology nurses play a vital role in facilitating education concerning the dangers of tobacco use, as well as advising survivors and their families about tobacco cessation. Oncology nurses are pivotal in advocating for tobacco control legislation to reduce the incidence of lung cancer. Lung cancer survivors face many challenges through the continuum of care that greatly impact QOL. Improved treatment modalities are a clinical priority to improve overall survival and QOL.

References

American Cancer Society. (2008). What are the key statistics about lung cancer? Retrieved November 6, 2008 from http://www.cdc.gov/cancer/lung/statistics/

Argiris, A., & Murren, J. R. (2001). Staging and clinical prognostic factors for small-cell lung cancer. *Cancer Journal*, 7(5), 437–444.

Brambilla, E., Travis, W. D., Colby, T. V., Corrin, B., & Shimosato, Y. (2001). The new world health organization classification of tumors. *European Respiratory Journal*, 18(6), 1059–1068.

Carney, D. N., & Hansen, H. H. (2000). Non-small cell lung cancer—stalemate or progress? *New England Journal of Medicine*, 343(17), 1261–1262.

Davies, M., Houlihan, N. G., & Joyce, M. (2004). Lung cancer control. In N. G. Houlihan (Ed.), *Lung cancer* (pp. 17–34). Pittsburgh, PA: Oncology Nursing Society.

Ettinger, D. S., & Aisner, J. (2006). Changing face of small-cell lung cancer: Real and artifact. *Journal of Clinical Oncology*, 24(28), 4526–4527.

Greene, F. L., Page, D. L., Fleming, I. D., Fritz, A., Balch, C. M., Haller, D. G., & Morrow, M. (Eds). (2002). *AJCC cancer staging manual* (6th ed.). New York: Springer.

Gritz, E. (2006). Smoking and smoking cessation in cancer patients. *Addiction*, 86(5), 549–554.

Houlihan, N. G. (2004). Overview. In N. G. Houlihan (Ed.), *Lung cancer* (pp. 1–6). Pittsburgh, PA: Oncology Nursing Society.

Houlihan, N. G., Inzeo, D., Joyce, M., & Tyson, L. B. (2004). Symptom management of lung cancer. In N. G. Houlihan (Ed.), *Lung cancer* (pp. 103–124). Pittsburgh, PA: Oncology Nursing Society.

Jemal, A., Thun, M. J., Ries, A. G., Howe, H. L., Weir, H. K., Center, M. M., *et al.* (2008). Annual report to the nation on the status of cancer, 1975–2005, featuring trends in lung cancer, tobacco use, and tobacco control. *Journal of the National Cancer Institute, 100*(23), 1672–1694.

Junker, K., Wiethege, T., & Muller, K. M. (2000). Pathology of small-cell lung cancer. *Journal of Cancer Research and Clinical Oncology, 126*(7), 1335–1432.

Joyce, M. (2004). Small cell lung cancer. In N. G. Houlihan (Ed.), *Lung cancer* (pp. 103–124). Pittsburgh, PA: Oncology Nursing.

McCormick, K. M. (2002). A concept analysis of uncertainty in illness. *Journal of Nursing Scholarship, 34*(2), 127–131.

Meert, A. P., Paesmans, M., Berghmans, T., Martin, B., Marcaux, C., Vallot, F., *et al.* (2001). Prophylactic cranial irradiation for patients with small cell lung cancer: A systematic review of the literature with meta analysis. BMC Cancer retrieved online March 3, 2009, from http://www.biomedcentral.com/1471–2407/1/5

Mountain, C. F. (1997). Revisions in the international system for staging lung cancer. *Chest, 111,* 1710–1717.

Mountain, C. F. (2000). International staging system for lung cancer. In H. I. Pass, J. B. Mitchell, D. H, Johnson, A. T. Turrisi, & J. D. Minna (Eds.), *Lung cancer: Principles and practice*. Philadelphia: Lippincott Williams & Wilkins.

National Cancer Institute. (2008). Retrieved November 6, 2008, from http://www.cancer.gov/Templates/db_alpha.aspx?CdrID=445089

National Comprehensive Cancer Network. (2009). Clinical practice guidelines in oncology: Non-small cell lung cancer. Retrieved March 3, 2009, from http://www.nccn.org/professionals/physician_gls/PDF/nscl.pdf

National Comprehensive Cancer Network. (2009). Clinical practice guidelines in oncology: Small cell lung cancer. Retrieved March 3, 2009, from http://www.nccn.org/professionals/physician_gls/PDF/sclc.pdf

Pignon, J. P., Tribodet H., Scagliotti, H., Douillard, J. Y., Shepard, F. A., Stephens, R. J., *et al.* (2008). Lung adjuvant evaluation: A pooled analysis by the LACE cooperative group. *Journal of Clinical Oncology, 26*(21), 3552–3559.

Sarna, L., Grannis, F. W., & Coscarelli, A. (2008). Physical and psychological issues in lung cancer survivorship. In P. A. Ganz (Ed.), *Cancer survivorship*. Los Angeles: Springer.

Taylor-Pilate, R. E., & Molassiotis, A. (2001). An exploration of the relationship between uncertainty, psychological distress and type of coping among Chinese men after cardiac catheterization. *Journal of Advanced Nursing, 33*(1), 70–88.

Travis, L. B., & Yahalom, J. (2008). Preface. In L. B. Travis & J. Yahalom (Eds.), *Cancer survivorship: Hematology / Oncology Clinics of North America*. Philadelphia: Saunders.

Tyson, L. B. (2004a). Non-small cell lung cancer. In N. G. Houlihan (Ed.), *Lung cancer* (pp. 103–124). Pittsburgh, PA: Oncology Nursing Society.

Tyson, L. B. (2004b). Paraneoplastic syndrome. In N. G. Houlihan (Ed.), *Lung cancer* (pp. 103–124). Pittsburgh, PA: Oncology Nursing Society.

Tyson, L. B. (2004). Oncologic urgencies and emergencies. In N. G. Houlihan (Ed.), *Lung cancer* (pp. 103–124). Pittsburgh, PA: Oncology Nursing Society.

World Health Organization (WHO). (2008). 10 facts on the tobacco epidemic and its control. Retrieved February 13, 2009, from http://www.who.int/features/factfiles/tobacco_epidemic/en/index.html

CHAPTER THREE

Follow Up and Surveillance: Screening, Testing, and Assessment

🎗 SCREENING

The overall poor survival of lung cancer survivors is attributable to the fact that the majority of patients have metastatic disease at the time of initial diagnosis. Historically, patients have been diagnosed following a work-up for symptoms suggestive of lung cancer or an incidental finding of a pulmonary lesion on a radiographic study conducted for another purpose, such as during the diagnostic work-up for pneumonia. Because of the high incidence of lung cancer, significant resources have been allocated for screening for early disease to improve the possibility of cure. Lung cancer accounts for 30% of deaths in the United States, with more than 160,000 deaths annually. For those individuals who undergo surgical resection, the survival rate is approximately 60% at 5 years (Mulshine, 2008).

There are certain characteristics of lung cancer that imply that screening for the disease would be beneficial: high morbidity and mortality; significant prevalence of 0.5–2.2%; known risk factors; and improved outcomes when therapy is initiated in early stage disease (Davies, Houlihan, & Joyce, 2004).

The goals of screening include the following (Henschke, Yankelevitz, Libby & Kimmel, 2002):

1. The search for asymptomatic individuals
2. Early diagnosis in order to apply effective early interventions, which incorporate specific regimens
3. Appropriate diagnostic measures and curability

Two main criteria are utilized to assess the benefit of screening. The screening test must *increase life expectancy* by early detection of disease so the usual course of the disease can be attenuated through treatment. The second criterion is that the test is *not painful or harmful* to the person or society. Direct harm to the person should not occur, nor should indirect harm from false-positives that can result in anxiety and unnecessary invasive and potentially dangerous procedures. The use of resources for screening must be appropriate and not impinge on the provision of care to others (Davies, Houlihan, & Joyce, 2004). The goal of utilizing a screening test in lung cancer is to identify individuals at increased risk for the disease. The ideal screening test would have high sensitivity and specificity, relative safety, be affordable, appeal to patients and healthcare providers, and reduce mortality and/or improve quality of life (Patz, Goodman, & Bepler, 2000).

The evidence that screening for lung cancer is beneficial is unclear and controversial. Because lung cancer is the leading cause of mortality in the United States and high-risk individuals can be readily identified by their smoking history and age, one would favor screening. The literature demonstrates that low-dose computed tomography (LDCT) is more sensitive than chest x-ray (CXR) in detecting lung cancer when the disease is small and the individual is asymptomatic. Unfortunately, detecting the disease earlier has not led to a reduction in mortality (Black, 2007). At this time the National Comprehensive

Cancer Network (NCCN) does not recommend screening for lung cancer (NCCN, 2009).

There are two important trials related to screening for lung cancer whose results have not yet been reported, but will be published in the near future and may provide answers related to the benefits of screening. The Prostate, Lung, Colorectal, and Ovarian (PCLO) cancer screening trial examined the cause-specific mortality reduction from screening for these four cancers in men and women. The second trial is the National Lung Cancer Screening Trial (NLST), a randomized controlled trial that evaluated whether there is a reduction in mortality by screening with LDCT (Black, 2007; Oken *et al.*, 2005).

Genetic Screening

There is a need for further research in genetics. Less than 20% of smokers develop lung cancer. In addition, first-degree relatives of individuals with lung cancer have a significantly increased chance of developing the disease if they also smoke. Research teams from MD Anderson Cancer Center, Johns Hopkins University, and the Institute for Cancer Research and the University of Cambridge in the United Kingdom have located two spots of genetic variations on chromosome 15. These two variants are single-nucleotide polymorphisms (SNPs). Individuals who have one or two copies of the SNPs have an increased risk of developing lung cancer if they smoke. The risk ranges from 28 to 81%. In the future we may be able to identify individuals at high risk for developing the disease (MD Anderson, 2008).

Assessment

Characteristically, lung cancer is asymptomatic in the early stages. Symptoms occur when the tumor is large enough to interfere with normal lung function or has spread to another part of the body and causes problems such as pain (Tyson, 2004). Once a tissue diagnosis of lung cancer has been established, patients undergo a series of tests to establish the stage of the disease. Local-regional symptoms related to the tumor are numerous. Cough is the most common symptom, occurring in 50–75% of lung cancer patients (Ingle, 2000; Tyson, 2004). Dyspnea is the second most common symptom, occurring in 40–60% of lung cancer patients (Tyson, 2004) (see section on Dyspnea in Chapter 4). In 30–50% of survivors, chest pain is a distressing symptom. It may be related to direct chest wall invasion or patients who have a superior sulcus tumor (apical tumor) that causes pain and numbness in the arm as the tumor grows. Pain needs immediate attention and treatment (Tyson, 2004; Warren, 2000) (see Chapter 4). Other local-regional symptoms include hemoptysis, stridor, hoarseness, hiccups, pneumonia, pleural effusion, superior vena cava syndrome, pericardial effusion atelectasis, Horner's syndrome, and bone pain (Ingle, 2000). When the tumor spreads out of the thorax it is called extrathoracic spread. The most common phenomenon is metastatic spread of the tumor to the brain, which occurs in up to 50% of individuals with small cell lung cancer (SCLC) and to a less degree in non-small cell lung cancer (NSCLC). Signs and symptoms are directly related to the location and amount of swelling. Other symptoms associated with this type of spread include gastrointestinal disturbances, jaundice, hepatomegaly, and abdominal pain. Systemic symptoms are not always present at diagnosis. The presentation is about the same for NSCLC and SCLC. Although the etiology is not always clearly understood, the systemic symptoms may include anorexia, fatigue, weakness, loss of weight, and/or symptoms associated with paraneoplastic syndromes (Ingle, 2000; Tyson, 2004).

It is necessary to have a tissue diagnosis in order to establish the type of lung cancer, as treatment differs for NSCLC and SCLC. A history and physical (H&P) is obtained. In addition, noninvasive diagnostic testing is conducted. Laboratory testing includes hematological and metabolic assessment: a complete blood count (CBC) and a comprehensive metabolic profile (CMP), which includes electrolytes and hepatic and renal function. The patient undergoes a computed tomography (CT) or positron emission tomography (PET) scan (AJCC, 2002). Magnetic resonance imaging (MRI) of the brain is indicated, especially if the patient has SCLC. The patient should receive smoking cessation counseling (NCCN, 2009). If the patient is a candidate for surgical resection, pretreatment evaluation includes the preceding as well as pulmonary function tests and possible mediastinoscopy. Other invasive diagnostic testing includes needle aspiration and bronchoscopy (NCCN, 2009).

Lung cancer survivors who are currently or were previously smokers are at risk for another primary cancer of the aerodigestive tract (e.g., head and neck cancers) and need to be evaluated frequently to detect recurrence of the development of a secondary malignancy. Long-term follow up includes a history and physical, contrast CT of the chest every 4–6 months for 2 years, and a noncontrast CT of the chest annually after 2 years. A PET scan may also be utilized (NCCN, 2009).

All lung cancer survivors should be encouraged to receive annual immunizations such as influenza vaccination and pneumococcal vaccination, if appropriate. Survivors need to have routine monitoring, including blood pressure, cholesterol and glucose monitoring, bone health, dental health, and routine sun protection. Survivors need to be encouraged to maintain a healthy weight, adopt an active lifestyle, consume a healthy diet, and limit alcohol consumption (NCCN, 2009). A screening tool that would enable lung cancer to be detected earlier with a decrease in mortality is paramount. Screening for tobacco use at every visit and aiding in the cessation of tobacco use is crucial to help halt this deadly disease.

References

Black, W. C. (2007). Computed tomography screening for lung cancer: Review of screening principles and update on current status. *Cancer, 110*(11), 2370–2384.

Davies, M., Houlihan, N. G., & Joyce, M. (2004). Lung cancer control. In N. G. Houlihan (Ed.), *Lung cancer* (pp. 17–34). Pittsburgh, PA: Oncology Nursing Society.

Henschke, C., Yankelevitz, D. F., Libby, D., & Kimmel, M. (2002). CT screening for lung cancer: The first 10 years. *The Cancer Journal, 8,* Suppl 1, s47–s54.

Ingle, R. J. (2000). Lung cancers. In C. H. Yarbro, M. H. Frogge, M. Goodman, & S. L. Groenwald (Eds.), *Cancer nursing: Principles and practice* (5th ed., pp. 1298–1328). Sudbury, MA: Jones and Bartlett.

MD Anderson Cancer Center. (2008). Genetic variations raise lung cancer risk for smokers and ex-smokers. Lung Cancer. Retrieved March 1, 2009, from http://www.eurekalert.org/pub_releases/2008-04/uotm-gvr033108.php

Mulshine, J. L. (2008). Current status of lung cancer screening. In H. Hansen (Ed.), *Textbook of lung cancer* (2nd ed., pp. 53–60). Copenhagen: Informa Healthcare.

National Comprehensive Cancer Network. (2009). Clinical practice guidelines in oncology: Non-small cell lung cancer. Retrieved March 3, 2009, from http://www.nccn.org/professionals/physician_gls/PDF/nscl.pdf

Oken, M. M., Beck, T. M., Hocking, W., Kvale, P. A., Cordes, J., Riley, T. L., *et al.* (2005). Baseline chest radiograph for lung cancer detection in a randomized prostate, lung, colorectal and ovarian cancer screening trial. *Journal of the National Cancer Institute, 97*(240), 1832–1839.

Patz, E. F., Goodman, P. C., & Bepler, G. (2000). Screening for lung cancer. *New England Journal of Medicine, 343*(22), 1627–1633.

Tyson, L. B. (2004). Non-small cell lung cancer. In N. G. Houlihan (Ed.), *Lung cancer* (pp. 103–124). Pittsburgh, PA: Oncology Nursing Society.

Warren, W. H. (2000). Chest wall involvement including Pancoast tumors. In H. I. Pass, J. B. Mitchell, D. H. Johnson, A. T. Turrisi, & J. D. Minna (Eds.), *Lung cancer: Principles and practice.* Philadelphia: Lippincott Williams & Wilkins.

❀ GENETIC COUNSELING
Kasia Bloch

❀ Introduction

Contrary to media portrayal of cancer and heredity, only approximately 5–10% of all types of cancer are hereditary in nature. Individuals with a hereditary predisposition to cancer have a significantly higher risk of developing cancer, typically multiple cancers, compared with those in the general population. For this reason, it is important to identify those individuals and their families who may be at risk and provide appropriate screening tests, prevention strategies, and management options. It is never too late to offer genetic counseling, the implications for those who already have had cancer are just as significant as for those relatives without any history of cancer. Even for cancer survivors, there is typically increased risk of other cancers.

❀ Cancer Genetics: The Basics

Many hereditary cancer syndromes have been identified to date. Most are autosomal dominant in nature, caused by tumor suppressor genes leading to the emergence of specific patterns when analyzing family histories. This section reviews some basic concepts in cancer genetics: autosomal dominant inheritance, tumor suppressor genes, and the patterns or *red flags*.

Autosomal-Dominant Inheritance

To review, genes are the blueprints for proteins that are crucial for normal development and function of our bodies, and they come in pairs.

One set is contributed from the mother and the other from the father. In autosomal dominant inheritance, the gene carrying a mutation is located on one of the autosomes (chromosome pairs 1–22), making it equally likely for a male or female offspring to inherit the mutation. Dominant means that having a mutation in just one of the two copies of a particular gene is enough to increase one's risk of developing cancer. When a parent has a dominant gene mutation, there is a 50% chance that each child will also inherit the mutation (Figure 3-1).

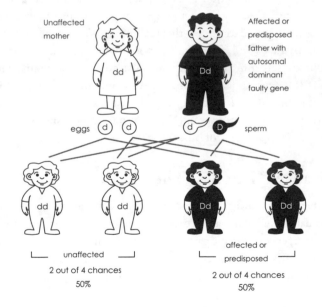

Figure 3-1   Autosomal Dominant Inheritance—Traditional Patterns of Inheritance 2. (From: Barlow-Stewart, K. (2007). *Autosomal dominant inheritance: Traditional patterns of inheritance 2*. Sydney: Centre for Genetics Education, Figure 9.1.)

Remember: Not everyone in a family with a hereditary predisposition to cancer will be at high risk.

Tumor Suppressor Genes

Tumor suppressor genes code for tumor suppressor proteins that, under normal conditions, act as "brakes" on cell growth. When these genes are missing or inactivated because of a mutation, the "brakes" fail and the cells can grow and divide out of control and may become malignant (American Society of Clinical Oncology [ASCO], 1998). Remember: Not everyone with a hereditary predisposition will acquire another mutation and develop cancer.

The Pattern or Red Flags

The presence of at least some of the features in the following list should raise the likelihood that cancer in the family may result from an inherited predisposition.

- Several relatives with same or related cancers, such as breast, ovarian and pancreatic cancers or colon, uterine, and ovarian cancers
- Younger age of onset than is typical, especially premenopausal breast cancer or colon cancer prior to the fifth decade
- Autosomal dominant pattern of inheritance
- Presence of rare cancers, such as men with breast cancer or non-smokers who develop early-onset lung cancer
- Excess of multifocal or bilateral cancers
- Excess of multiple primary cancers
- Presence of other nonmalignant features; for example, congenital hypertrophy of the retinal pigment epithelium (CHRPE), a distinctive eye finding associated with familial adenomatous polyposis (FAP)

- Absence of environmental risk factors; for example, lymphoma and Kaposi sarcoma in HIV-positive individuals or colon cancer in those with ulcerative colitis

✤ Genetic Counseling Process

The genetic counseling process is complex. Because decisions regarding genetic testing, screening, and prevention are based on the patterns described in the preceding paragraphs it is crucial to collect a detailed, three-generational family history to construct a pedigree. A pedigree is a diagram showing the ancestral relationships and transmission of genetic traits over at least three generations in a family. Sometimes medical records and death certificates may be obtained to verify a questionable history. Subsequently, the pedigree is analyzed using risk assessment models to assess one's risk of having a hereditary predisposition to cancer.

If the genetic risk is significant, the most appropriate person for genetic testing is identified in the family. It is typically encouraged that one begins by testing a family member who has had cancer or relatives who are most closely related to those with cancer history. The closest relative or the cancer survivor provides information as to whether a causative gene mutation can be identified in the family using current laboratory techniques. Unfortunately, most genetic tests are not 100% sensitive.

There are risks, benefits, and limitations of genetic testing and its implications for the test results. Psychological issues, as well as support systems, are explored to ensure that one is prepared for all the possible outcomes. Other questions about test cost coverage and genetic discrimination are addressed prior to testing. Over the last 5 years, there has been a significant increase in coverage for genetic testing by health insurance companies. In fact, most insurance companies have some, if not complete, coverage for genetic testing.

State laws addressing genetic discrimination have been in existence for the last 5–10 years. Currently, no cases have gone to court. In May 2008, the Genetic Information Nondiscrimination Act (GINA) was signed into law. This federal law, which went into effect in May 2009, protects individuals undergoing genetic testing from discrimination by health insurance companies and employers because of their genetic test results. Unfortunately, at this time, the same protections do not exist for life insurance or long-term care insurance.

Most genetic tests are simple blood draws, with results available in a couple of weeks to a couple of months. When the results are available, a test result disclosure appointment is set up with a genetic counselor. During this appointment, the genetic counselor provides an individual with his or her test result, along with a review of its implications for the person and his or her family. A screening, prevention, and management plan is designed that best suits the individual and ways of sharing this information with other family members are discussed. Finally, information on local, national, and worldwide research studies, as well as support groups, is provided.

☙ Summary

Cancer genetics is a fast-changing field. A good experience with the cancer genetic counseling process can make all the difference for survivors and their families. Oncology nurses can identify people with cancer who may have familial cancers to genetic counselors. Genetic counselors can be located through the National Society of Genetic Counselors (Table 3-1).

TABLE 3-1   Most Common Hereditary Cancer Syndromes

Syndrome (OMIM entry)	Component tumors	Mode of inheritance	Genes
Hereditary breast cancer syndromes			
Hereditary breast cancer and ovarian cancer syndrome (113705, 600185)	Breast cancer Ovarian cancer Prostate cancer Pancreatic cancer	Dominant	BRCA1 BRCA2
	Fanconi anemia/ medulloblastoma	Recessive	BRCA2
Li-Fraumeni syndrome (151623)	Soft tissue sarcoma Breast cancer Osteosarcoma Leukemia Brain tumors Adrenocortical carcinoma	Dominant	p53 CHEK2
Cowden syndrome (158350)	Breast cancer Thyroid cancer Endometrial and other cancers	Dominant	PTEN
Bannayan-Riley-Ruvalcaba syndrome (153480)	Breast cancer Meningioma Thyroid follicular cell tumors	Dominant	PTEN
Ataxia telangiectasia (208900)	Leukemia Lymphoma	Recessive	ATM

TABLE 3-1 (continued)

Hereditary gastrointestinal malignancies

HNPCC, including "Lynch II" syndrome (120435, 120436, 114500, 114400)	Colon cancer Endometrial cancer Ovarian cancer Renal pelvis cancers Ureteral cancers Pancreatic cancer Stomach and small bowel cancers Hepatobiliary cancers	Dominant	MLH1 MSH2 MSH6
Familial polyposis, including attenuated phenotype (175100)		Dominant	APC
Familial attenuated polyposis (175100)	Colon cancer	Dominant	APC
Hereditary gastric cancer (137215)	Stomach cancers	Dominant	CDH1
Juvenile polyposis (174900)	Gastrointestinal cancers Pancreatic cancer	Dominant	SMAD4/ DPC4 BMPR1A
Peutz-Jeghers syndrome (175200)	Colon cancer Small bowel cancer Breast cancer Ovarian cancer Pancreatic cancer	Dominant	STK11
Hereditary melanoma pancreatic cancer syndrome (606719)	Pancreatic cancer Melanoma	Dominant	CDKN2A/ p16

(continued)

TABLE 3-1   (continued)

Syndrome (OMIM entry)	Component tumors	Mode of inheritance	Genes
Hereditary pancreatitis (167800)	Pancreatic cancer	Dominant	PRSS1
Turcot syndrome (276300)	Colon cancer Basal cell carcinoma Ependymoma Medulloblastoma Glioblastoma	Dominant	APC MLH1 PMS2
Familial gastrointestinal stromal tumor (606764)	Gastrointestinal stromal tumors	Dominant	KIT
Genodermatoses with cancer predisposition			
Melanoma syndromes (155600, 155601, 609048, 608035)	Malignant melanoma	Dominant	CDKN2 (p16) CDK4 CMM
Basal cell cancers, Gorlin syndrome (109400)	Basal cell cancers Brain tumors	Dominant	PTCH
Cowden syndrome	See above	Dominant	PTEN
Neurofibromatosis 1 (162200)	Neurofibrosarcomas Pheochromocytomas Optic gliomas Meningiomas	Dominant	NF1
Neurofibromatosis 2 (101000)	Vestibular schwannomas	Dominant	NF2

TABLE 3-1   (continued)

Tuberous sclerosis (191100)	Myocardial rhabdomyoma	Dominant	TSC1
	Multiple bilateral renal angiomyolipoma		TSC2
	Ependymoma		
	Renal cancer		
	Giant cell astrocytoma		
Carney complex (160980, 605244)	Myxoid subcutaneous tumors	Dominant	PRKAR1A
	Primary adrenocortical nodular hyperplasia		
	Testicular Sertoli cell tumor		
	Atrial myxoma		
	Pituitary adenoma		
	Mammary fibroadenoma		
	Thyroid carcinoma		
	Schwannoma		
Muir-Torre syndrome (158320)	Sebaceous carcinoma	Dominant	MLH1
	Sebaceous epitheliomas		MSH2
	Sebaceous adenomas		
	Keratoacanthomas		
	Colon cancer		
	Laryngeal carcinoma		
	Malignant gastrointestinal tract tumors		
	Malignant genitourinary tract tumors		

(continued)

TABLE 3-1   (continued)

Syndrome (OMIM entry)	Component tumors	Mode of inheritance	Genes
Xeroderma pigmentosum (278730, 278700, 278720, 278760, 74740, 278780, 278750, 133510)	Skin cancer Melanoma Leukemia	Recessive	XPA,B,C,D, E,F,G POLH
Rothmund-Thomson syndrome (268400)	Basal cell carcinoma Squamous cell carcinoma Osteogenic sarcoma	Recessive	RECQL4
Leukemia/lymphoma predisposition syndromes			
Bloom syndrome (210900)	Leukemia Carcinoma of the tongue Squamous cancers Wilms' tumor Colon cancer	Recessive	BLM
Fanconi anemia (227650)	Leukemia Squamous cancers Skin carcinoma Hepatoma	Recessive	FANCA,B,C FANCA,D2 FANCE,F,G FANCL
Shwachman-Diamond syndrome (260400)	Myelodysplasia Acute myelogenous leukemia	Recessive	SBDS
Nijmegen breakage syndrome (251260)	Lymphoma Glioma Medulloblastoma Rhabdomyosarcoma	Recessive	NBS1

TABLE 3-1 (continued)

Canale-Smith syndrome (601859)	Lymphoma	Dominant	FAS FASL

Immunodeficiency syndromes

Wiskott-Aldrich syndrome (301000)	Hematopoietic malignancies	X-linked recessive	WAS
Common variable immune deficiency (240500)	Lymphomas	Recessive Dominant	Unknown Unknown
Severe combined immune deficiency (102700, 300400, 312863, 601457, 600802, 602450)	B-cell lymphoma	X-linked recessive Recessive	IL2RG ADA JAK3 RAG1 RAG2 IL7R CD45 Artemis
X-linked lymphoproliferative syndrome (308240)	Lymphoma	X-linked recessive	SH2D1A

Genitourinary cancer predisposition syndromes

Hereditary prostate cancer (176807, 601518)	Prostate cancer	Dominant	HPC1 HPCX HPC2/ ELAC2 PCAP PCBC PRCA

(continued)

TABLE 3-1 (continued)

Syndrome (OMIM entry)	Component tumors	Mode of inheritance	Genes
Simpson-Golabi-Behmel syndrome (312870)	Embryonal tumors Wilms' tumor	X-linked recessive	GPC3
von Hippel-Lindau syndrome (193300)	Hemangioblastomas of retina and central nervous system Renal cell cancer Pheochromocytomas	Dominant	VHL
Beckwith-Wiedemann syndrome (130650)	Wilms' tumor Hepatoblastoma Adrenal carcinoma Gonadoblastoma	Dominant	CDKN1C NSD1
Wilms' tumor syndrome (194070)	Wilms' tumor	Dominant	WT1
WAGR: Wilms' tumor, aniridia, genitourinary abnormalities, mental retardation (194072)	Wilms' tumor Gonadoblastoma	Dominant	WT1
Birt-Hogg-Dubé syndrome (135150)	Renal tumors	Dominant	FLCL
Papillary renal cancer syndrome (605074)	Papillary renal cancer	Dominant	MET, PRCC

TABLE 3-1   (continued)

Constitutional t(3;8) translocation (603046)	Renal cell cancer	Dominant	TRC8
Hereditary bladder cancer (109800)	Bladder cancer	Sporadic Unknown	Unknown
Hereditary testicular cancer (273300)	Testicular cancer	Possibly X-linked Possibly recessive	Unknown Unknown
Rhabdoid predisposition syndrome (601607)	Rhabdoid tumors (see below)	Dominant	SNF5/INI1
Central nervous system/vascular cancer predisposition syndromes			
Hereditary paraganglioma (185470, 115310, 16800)	Paraganglioma Pheochromocytoma	Dominant	SDHD SDHC SDHB
Retinoblastoma (180200)	Retinoblastoma Osteosarcoma	Dominant	RB1
Rhabdoid predisposition syndrome (601607)	Rhabdoid tumors Medulloblastoma Choroid plexus tumors Primitive neuroectodermal tumors	Dominant	SNF5/INI1

(continued)

TABLE 3-1 (continued)

Syndrome (OMIM entry)	Component tumors	Mode of inheritance	Genes
Sarcoma/bone cancer predisposition syndromes			
Multiple exostoses (133700, 133701)	Chondrosarcoma	Dominant	EXT1 EXT2
Leiomyoma/renal cancer syndrome (605839)	Papillary renal cell carcinoma Uterine leiomyosarcomas	Dominant	FH
Carney complex	See above	Dominant	PRKAR1A
Werner syndrome (277700)	Sarcoma/osteosarcoma Meningioma	Recessive	WRN
Endocrine cancer predisposition syndromes			
MEN1 (131100)	Pancreatic islet cell tumors Pituitary adenomas Parathyroid adenomas	Dominant	MEN1
MEN2 (171400)	Medullary thyroid cancers Pheochromocytoma Parathyroid hyperplasia	Dominant	RET
Familial papillary thyroid cancer (188500)	Papillary thyroid cancer	Dominant	Multiple loci

Abbreviations: HNPCC, hereditary nonpolyposis colorectal cancer; MEN, multiple endocrine neoplasia; OMIM, ON-LINE Mendelian Inheritance in Man.

From: Garber & Offit, 2005, Table 2.

Genetic Risk and Lung Cancer

Lung cancer is a relatively common disease within the general population, especially in present or past smokers. Only a small percentage of lung cancer is caused by inherited alterations in cancer susceptibility genes. There are no cancer susceptibility genes that have been identified to date involved in hereditary cancer predisposition conditions or syndromes associated with a higher risk of lung cancer. However, there is ongoing research in the field of lung cancer that is looking to identify susceptibility genes for lung cancer. Families who are eligible are encouraged to participate in studies including those with patterns consistent with hereditary predisposition to lung cancer based on their family histories. These include families with multiple relatives with lung cancer, especially those diagnosed at a young age and/or lacking exposure to environmental risk factors such as smoking.

Genetic Tests: Tumors and Targeted Therapy

New genetic testing of tumors allows for the oncologists to determine the best chemotherapy. This is especially true in colorectal cancer, in which KRAS mutation testing refers to testing the tumor itself. KRAS mutation is an acquired mutation (during tumorigenesis), not an inherited one. It helps to predict response to chemotherapy. The mutations occur on the codons (triplets of nucleotides on the DNA) 12 and 13 and predict lack of response to antibodies targeted to the epidermal growth factor receptor, such as cetuximab (Erbitux).

References

ASCO Curriculum (1998). Cancer Genetics & Cancer Predisposition Testing [PowerPoint slides].

Barlow-Stewart, K. (2007). Autosomal dominant inheritance—traditional patterns of inheritance 2. Centre for Genetics Education. Retrieved February 14, 2009, from http://www.genetics.com.au/factsheet/fs9.html

Garber, J. E., & Offit, K. (2005). Hereditary cancer predisposition syndromes. *Journal of Clinical Oncology, 23,* 278–280.

Bibliography

Schneider, K. (2002). *Counseling about cancer: Strategies for genetic counseling.* New York: Wiley-Liss, Inc.

Resources

ClinicalTrials.gov: http://www.clinicaltrials.gov/
   A registry of federally and privately supported clinical trials conducted in the United States and around the world, including research studies for individuals with a hereditary predisposition to cancer

(FORCE) Facing Our Risk of Cancer Empowered: http://www.facingourrisk.org/
   Online support organization for individuals at high risk for breast and ovarian cancer started by a woman with a BRCA2 mutation

GeneTests: http://www.genetests.org/
   Web site where you can find detailed overviews of the common hereditary cancer syndromes, including information about risks, management, and genetic testing

National Conference of State Legislatures: http://www.ncsl.org/programs/health/genetics/charts.htm
   Web site that provides detailed information on existing state laws regarding genetic discrimination as related to health insurance, employment, life, disability and long-term care insurance, etc.

National Human Genome Research Institute: http://www.genome.gov/10002328
   Web site that provides and answers basic information and questions about GINA, including a link to the text of the bill

National Society of Genetic Counselors: www.nsgc.org
   Web site where you can find additional information about cancer genetics and genetic counseling, as well as a search engine to find a genetic counselor in your area

Interventions for Side Effects of Cancer and Its Treatment

🎗 Introduction

Treatment of cancer can affect many body systems while targeting the specific malignancy. Although acute side effects develop during treatment, many long-term effects of treatment develop years later. For example, lymphedema after breast cancer treatment may develop years after the initial surgery. Diarrhea from radiation enteritis may afflict survivors previously treated with radiation to the pelvis and abdomen years after the treatment. Oncology nurses continue to monitor and assess cancer survivors based on an understanding of the cancer, the treatment, and the potential for ongoing issues, years after treatment. This section covers the interventions for common side effects of cancer and its treatment, including:

- Bowel dysfunction
- Pain
- Fatigue
- Peripheral neuropathy
- Anxiety

- Depression
- Sleep disturbances
- Cultural awareness
- Dyspnea
- Cognitive dysfunction
- Sexuality

❦ BOWEL DYSFUNCTION

Lisa Kennedy Sheldon

❦ Introduction

Bowel dysfunction is a common side effect of cancer treatments. Changes in bowel functioning may range from diarrhea to constipation, fecal leakage and incontinence, to ostomy creation. Changes in bowel functioning have important implications for survivors because they may affect body image, functioning in social roles and intimate relationships, and overall quality of life (QOL). Nurses are frequently the source of information for survivors because of their ability to address these concerns and their knowledge about interventions to prevent changes, manage alterations, and improve bowel functioning.

❦ Diarrhea

According to the Oncology Nursing Society's (ONS) Putting Evidence into Practice® (PEP) Team, diarrhea is defined as "an abnormal increase in stool liquidity, frequency ($\geq$4–6 stools/day over baseline) with or without nocturnal bowel movements." It may develop as a result of treatment such as chemotherapy with irinotecan (Camptosar) or as a result of radiation therapy to the abdomen and pelvis for colorectal or prostate cancers, and may cause diarrhea both during and after treatment.

Oncology nurses should carefully assess for changes in bowel functioning that may be defined as diarrhea because increased frequency of stools can be caused by a number of factors. For example, diarrhea may be caused by *salmonella, clostridium difficile, escherichia coli, campylobacter,* and other types of infectious colitis. Ongoing diarrhea may also cause dehydration, weakness, hypotension, tachycardia, and electrolyte imbalances.

TABLE 4-1   Prevention and Treatment of Diarrhea

Medication	Dosage	Notes
Loperamide	Initial dose: 4 mg Subsequent doses: 2 mg every 4 hours or after every unformed stool	First line for chemotherapy induced diarrhea May be given high dose (2 mg every 2 hours) for 48 hours for irinotecan-induced diarrhea
Diphenoxylate	2 tabs 4 times/day 10 ml 4 times/day (20 mg/day)	
Probiotics *Lactobacillus acidophilus* *Lactobacillus rhamnosus*		Supplementation during/2 weeks after radiation
Psyllium fiber	1–2 teaspoons/day orally	Supplementation during pelvic radiation
Octreotide acetate	100 mcg SC 3 times/day	
Neomycin	660 mg orally 3 times/day	Begin 2 days before irinotecan
Amifostine	800 mg/m^2 IV	Used during 5-fluorouracil infusions

Source: Putting Evidence into Practice: Evidence Based Interventions to Prevent, Manage and Treat Chemotherapy or Radiation Therapy Induced Diarrhea, by Paula Muehlbauer, Deborah Thorpe, Arlene Davis, Rachael Drabot, Barbara Rawlings, and Elizabeth Kiker, (in press), Clinical Journal of Oncology Nursing, 13(3). Copyright 2009 by the Oncology Nursing Society. Adapted with permission

Treatment for diarrhea depends on the cause and severity of the symptom experience. Because diarrhea may be accompanied by painful cramping and may cause dehydration, prevention and early treatment are important components of oncology care. Increasingly, radiation-induced diarrhea is being treated prophylactically with probiotic and psyllium oral supplementation (ONS, 2008). Treatment of radiation-induced diarrhea is managed with oral opiates such as loperamide and diphenoxylate, and prophylactic treatment with probiotics and psyllium may also be recommended (Table 4-1).

Constipation

Constipation is a common problem for many cancer survivors. It may result from dehydration, opioids for pain relief, decreased intake of fiber, or vinca alkaloid chemotherapeutic agents such as vincristine. Because it is often multifactorial, a holistic approach to the experience of constipation is necessary. A thorough history provides information on bowel functioning, medications, and dietary habits. A nutritional consult may also be helpful in assessing dietary intake. A more in-depth evaluation may be needed if initial interventions are not effective, because some physiologic and anatomic issues, such as bowel obstructions, may cause constipation, cramping, and discomfort.

Prevention of constipation is the most effective measure to improve bowel functioning. Survivors should be encouraged to have a diet high in fiber and sufficient liquids (eight 8-oz. glasses per day). If medications that are known to slow colonic transit times, such as prescribed opioids, are prescribed, then the patient may need prophylactic stool softeners and stimulant laxatives (docusate sodium and senna). Stronger medications, such as polyethylene glycol and lactulose, may be needed for

TABLE 4-2   Medication to Prevent and Treat Constipation

Medication	Dosage	Notes
Docusate sodium	100–300 mg/day orally	May be combined with senna to prevent opioid-induced constipation
Senna	2–6 tablets/twice a day	May be combined with docusate sodium to prevent opioid-induced constipation
Psyllium Methylcellulose	1–2 teaspoons/day	Bulk laxatives are not recommended for opioid-induced constipation or in dehydrated patients.
Polyethelene glycol (PEG) PEG 3350 Miralax GoLYTELY Colyte	Dosages vary	May be used to treat refractory constipation
Glycerin suppositories	One per rectum	
Mineral oil	15–30 ml orally 1–2 times/day	Lubricant and stool softener
Osmotic laxatives: Sorbitol Lactulose	Dosage varies	Used in combination with stimulant laxatives in refractory constipation
Castor oil	15–30 ml orally	Not recommended because of cramping
Bisacodyl	1–2 tablets orally at bedtime	Stimulant laxative; Not studied in oncology patients
Magnesium salts Milk of Magnesia	15–30 ml orally once a day	

refractory constipation or no bowel movement in 3 days with the use of a bowel regimen. Constipation with impaction may require suppositories, enemas, and/or manual disimpaction (Table 4-2).

Prevention is the most important way to avoid constipation. Oncology nurses can teach survivors to increase dietary fiber, maintain an adequate intake of liquids, and begin a bowel regimen when potentially constipating medications are being taken. Laxative doses should be titrated for the individual person with parameters; for example, use lactulose if there is no bowel movement after 3 days while taking stool softeners and stimulants. Treating constipation in myelosuppressed people requires more care. Manual disimpaction should be avoided. Manipulation of the stoma in myelosuppressed patients or those with neutropenia should also be avoided. Preventive regimens are important to maintain regularity and consistency and decrease the likelihood of passage of hard stool that could cause anal fissures.

References

Oncology Nursing Society's Putting Evidence into Practice (PEP) Team. (2008). Constipation. Retrieved February 10, 2009, from http://www.ons.org/outcomes/volume2/constipation.shtml

PAIN
Jeannine M. Brant

Introduction

Pain is a common problem in patients with cancer. Approximately 50% of patients experience pain in the earlier stages of the disease, and about 75% have pain with advanced disease. More recent studies reveal that pain can also become chronic and linger beyond the treatment phase, thus affecting posttreatment cancer survivors. Chronic pain in cancer survivors has not been well studied, and the prevalence is unknown. In addition, the problem may be underappreciated by both patients and healthcare professionals when compared with surviving cancer. Unfortunately, chronic pain can lead to depression, anxiety, sleep disturbance, functional deficits, and poor QOL.

This chapter provides an overview of the various types of chronic pain that can occur in cancer survivors, discusses pain assessment parameters in cancer survivors, and outlines global treatment strategies to manage pain and optimize QOL.

Types of Pain Syndromes in Cancer Survivors

Pain in cancer survivors may be related to residual effects from the tumor but is most commonly a consequence of cancer treatment. The trajectory of pain can vary with some pain syndromes beginning at the time of diagnosis, some after cancer treatment, and others up to 20 years after initial treatment. Specific pain syndromes are identified in the following section.

Postsurgical Pain

Surgery is a primary treatment modality for many types of cancer. Acute pain is a normal postsurgical outcome, but pain can persist beyond normal healing and become chronic over time. Overall predictors of chronic postsurgical pain include poor control of acute postsurgical pain, radiation and/or chemotherapy after surgery, and anxiety and depression. Limb amputation, mastectomy, thoracotomy, and head and neck surgery are some of the most common types of cancer surgeries that may cause chronic pain.

Limb Amputation

Amputation of an extremity is a common treatment modality in patients with osteosarcoma. Limb amputation results in two types of pain: stump pain and phantom limb pain (PLP). Stump pain can be described as aching, sore, swollen, shooting, or numb, and involves nociceptive (myofascial and soft tissue) and neuropathic components. Poorly fitting prostheses can contribute to unrelieved pain. Phantom pain, mediated by the central nervous system, is often described as neuropathic pain (shooting, numbness, burning, tingling, pins and needles sensation) sensed in the location of the absent limb. Up to 72% of patients continue to suffer PLP 6 months after amputation, and 5–10% go on to experience chronic, persistent pain. Risk factors for chronic PLP include female gender, severe postoperative pain, pain present 1 year after amputation, a more proximal amputation, and adjuvant chemotherapy. Anticonvulsants, antidepressants, and other adjuvant analgesics are sometimes effective in relieving the pain.

Breast Cancer Surgery

Mastectomy, the primary treatment for breast cancer, may cause phantom breast pain or neuropathic pain in up to 50% of patients.

Postmastectomy pain syndrome (PMPS) is thought to be related to trauma of the intercostobrachial nerve. Patients commonly describe the pain as burning, shooting, electric shock-like, or hypersensitive. Pain can involve the neck, arm, axilla, scar, or chest wall and can contribute to functional deficits. Specifically, patients may limit range of motion to prevent pain and can develop a "frozen shoulder". Possible risk factors for the development of PMPS include younger age, obesity, and extensive axillary dissection. Topical analgesics and adjuvants are common strategies to manage pain; opioids are used less often.

Thoracotomy

Thoracotomy is a common surgical intervention for non-small cell lung cancer. Up to 60% of patients may suffer from chronic postthoracotomy pain 1 year postoperatively, and about 5% report the pain as severe and disabling. Risk factors for chronic pain include lack of optimal postoperative pain and a possible slight increase in pain with open thoracotomy compared with less invasive video-assisted surgery. Postoperative pain primarily occurs along the surgical scar and is related to intercostal nerve injury. The pain is often described as moderate to severe and includes aching or neuropathic sensations. Some patients can also develop myofascial pain because of immobility and frozen shoulder syndrome. Analgesics and intercostal nerve blockade are mainstay therapies.

Head and Neck Cancer Surgery

Surgery for head and neck cancer can cause pain because of injury to the accessory nerve and superficial cervical plexus nerves. About 40% of patients continue to complain of pain 1 year after surgery and about 15% at 5 years. Pain can be described as both nociceptive and neuropathic. Pain commonly extends down the shoulder and contributes to functional disabilities. The degree of disability correlated significantly with severe pain. Early shoulder and neck mobility may potentially decrease the incidence of chronic pain.

Pain Related to Chemotherapy

Chemotherapy-induced peripheral neuropathy (CIPN) is a growing problem among cancer survivors. Novel chemotherapy agents have led to an increase in response rates, but many of these newer agents can induce nerve damage and cause chronic pain and functional deficits. Several classes of chemotherapy contribute to CIPN, including the taxanes, plant alkaloids, platinum-based compounds, epothilone, thalidomide, and bortezomib. Some antimitotics such as methotrexate, fluorouracil, and cytosine arabinoside have also been shown to cause CIPN. Risk factors for the development of CIPN include younger age, preexisting neuropathies such as diabetic neuropathy, high-dose chemotherapy, receiving multiple agents that cause CIPN, alcohol abuse, and genetic predisposition (see section on Peripheral Neuropathy, page 63).

The sensorimotor pain syndrome that occurs in a "stocking-and-glove" distribution can be described as progressive numbness, tingling, and motor dysfunction after chemotherapy administration. Pain and motor dysfunction may become cumulative over time, and dose reduction is often employed to ameliorate the symptoms. The onset and course of the pain varies for each agent. For some patients, neurotoxicity disappears over time, but some cancer survivors experience persistent discomfort or pain years after the completion of treatment. Studies are underway to investigate methods to prevent and ameliorate CIPN.

Pain Related to Radiation Therapy

Radiation-related pain syndromes are caused by damage to nerves or tissue after radiation treatment. Fortunately, advances in radiation therapy have significantly decreased the incidence of these painful syndromes.

Radiation-induced pain is usually a late effect of treatment with some radiation-induced injuries, such as myelopathy, presenting months or even years after treatment. The types of pain syndromes exhibited vary according to the location of the radiation field. Brachial plexopathy occurs following radiation therapy to the chest or breast. Initial symptoms are described as dysesthetic sensations in the shoulder and down the affected arm with progression to pain and limb weakness. High-dose radiation therapy is strongly correlated with the development of brachial plexopathy. Chronic pelvic pain has also been described in the literature following pelvic radiation for prostate cancer, endometrial cancer, and cervical cancer. Because of the delay in symptoms, clinicians should be on alert for these radiation-induced pain syndromes, even years after treatment.

Tumor-Related Pain

The least common type of pain in cancer survivors involves infiltration of nerves, tissue, or bone caused by the original tumor. Occasionally, patients may achieve a complete response or even cure from cancer therapy but be left from residual tumor-related pain that occurred prior to treatment. For example, a patient with testicular cancer may have extensive disease including invasion of bone into the spinal nerves at diagnosis. Although the patient may be cured with chemotherapy, he may be left with chronic neuropathic pain resulting from permanent nerve damage. Treatment is individualized according to the specific pain syndrome exhibited.

✤ Pain Assessment in Cancer Survivors

Clinicians should be alert for pain syndromes that affect cancer survivors and should conduct a comprehensive pain assessment on all patients with a history of cancer. It is important to recognize that pain syndromes can occur at diagnosis, during or immediately after treatment, or months or years into survivorship. If pain is present, then depression, fatigue, and

---

TABLE 4-3   Pain Assessment Parameters in Cancer Survivors

Assess Cancer History

Location of cancer
Metastatic disease sites
Pain at disease presentation

Assess Cancer Treatment History

Surgical interventions: Type of surgery, extent of surgery, postoperative
recovery (postoperative pain intensity, complications)
Radiation therapy: Year treated, fields treated, dose, immediate side effects
Chemotherapy: Types of chemotherapy, doses, immediate side effects

If Pain Is Present

Location: May be more than one location of pain
Intensity: 0–10 scale with 0 being no pain and 10 being worst possible pain
Quality: Describe the pain
Temporal factors: Onset, duration, pattern, alleviating factors,
exacerbating factors
Function: Ability to work, activities of daily living, functional deficits
Interventions: Pharmacologic and nonpharmacologic interventions tried to
alleviate the pain
Associated symptoms: Depression, fatigue, sleep disturbance

---

sleep disturbance should be assessed, as they often coexist with pain. An overview of pain assessment parameters is included in Table 4-3. Optimal assessment leads to tailored pain management interventions that can alleviate pain and associated symptoms and improve QOL.

❀ Management of Pain in Cancer Survivors

Early detection and prompt management of acute pain at diagnosis and during cancer treatment is paramount in the prevention of chronic, persistent pain in cancer survivors. For example, for many postoperative pain syndromes, poor postoperative control is a risk factor in the development of chronic pain. For CIPN, early detection of pain can lead to dose reduction and can lessen nerve damage and chronic pain.

Early mobility is another important front-line intervention in the prevention of chronic pain. Neck, arm, and shoulder mobility is essential for patients undergoing mastectomy, thoracotomy, and head and neck surgeries. Immobility can lead to myofascial pain syndromes, including frozen shoulder.

When pain persists beyond healing in cancer survivors, interventions should be employed at alleviating pain, improving function, and enhancing QOL. Nonpharmacologic interventions include nerve blocks for pain syndromes such as thoracotomy and other postoperative pain syndromes. Adjuvants are a mainstay treatment for neuropathic pain, including PMPS and CIPN. Adjuvants include tricyclic antidepressants (amitriptyline, desipramine, nortriptyline), serotonin nonspecific reuptake inhibitors (venlafaxine, duloxetine), anticonvulsants (gabapentin, pregabalin, lamotrigine, clonazepam), local anesthetics (mexiletine), alpha-2 adrenergic agonists (tizanidine, clonidine), NMDA antagonists (ketamine, dextromethorphan), and topical agents (capsaicin, local anesthetic creams). First-line therapy for neuropathic pain is gabapentin followed by other adjuvant therapies previously listed. When pain is severe and uncontrolled with adjuvant agents, opioids can be used in select patients. Long-acting opioids are recommended for constant pain with breakthrough dosing of short-acting opioids for acute exacerbations of pain. Patients receiving opioids require a bowel protocol to prevent constipation. Occasionally, more invasive routes of pain control are used such as nerve stimulators and implantable pumps that deliver opioid and local anesthetic agents at the spinal level. Overall, treatment should be individualized according to pain intensity, functional status, and tolerance of the selected regimen.

❀ Summary

Advances in cancer treatment have led to long-term survival in many tumor types. Cure rates and life expectancy have increased dramatically, and cancer is becoming a chronic disease that is controlled long term. However, surviving cancer can be difficult if the patient is left with long-term sequelae from the disease and/or cancer treatment, such as chronic pain. Therefore, clinicians should be on alert to: (1) aggressively control acute cancer and treatment-related pain to prevent the development of chronic pain, (2) conduct a comprehensive pain assessment on all cancer survivors, and (3) develop an optimal pain management plan for cancer survivors whose pain persists beyond the normal healing time. Overall, adequate pain control can enhance the physical and psychosocial well-being of the cancer survivor.

Bibliography

Aziz, N. M. (2007). Cancer survivorship research: State of knowledge, challenges and opportunities. *Acta Oncologica, 46*(4), 417–432.

Burton, A. W., Fanciullo, G. J., Beasley, R. D., & Fisch, M. J. (2007). Chronic pain in the cancer survivor: A new frontier. *Pain Medicine, 8*(2), 189–198.

Cancer Care. (2009). Accessed January 9, 2009, from http://www.cancercare.org/get_help/special_progs/post_treatment.php

Ferrell, B., Paice, J., & Koczywas, M. (2008). New standards and implications for improving the quality of supportive oncology practice. *Journal of Clinical Oncology, 26*(23), 3824–3831.

National Cancer Comprehensive Network. (2008). Adult Cancer Pain Guidelines. Retrieved January 12, 2009, from http://www.nccn.org/professionals/physician_gls/PDF/pain.pdf

Polomano, R. C., & Farrar, J. T. (2006). Pain and neuropathy in cancer survivors. *Cancer Nursing, 29*(2), 39–47.

Saxena, A. K., & Kumar, S. (2007). Management strategies for pain in breast carcinoma patients: Current opinions and future perspectives. *Pain Practice, 7*(2), 163–177.

FATIGUE AND SURVIVORSHIP

Lisa Kennedy Sheldon

Introduction

The experience of fatigue has important ramifications for the QOL for cancer survivors (Mock, 2004; Nail, 2002, 2004). Fatigue can affect physical and psychosocial functioning and have a significant impact on symptom distress and QOL (Mitchell, Beck, Hood, Moore, & Tanner, 2007). Once initial treatment is completed, many survivors are tired and lack the energy to continue or resume their normal activities.

Assessment

Fatigue has been defined as a persistent and subjective sense of tiredness that interferes with usual functioning (Mock, 2004). Understanding the exact nature of the experience of fatigue helps to identify and implement the appropriate interventions. Olson (2007) described the experience of fatigue as having three components: tiredness, fatigue, and exhaustion.

- *Tiredness* is characterized by forgetfulness, impatience, gradual weakness in muscles after work, and sleepiness relieved by rest.
- *Fatigue* is characterized by difficulty concentrating, anxiety, decreased stamina out of proportion to energy used, difficulty sleeping, increased sensitivity to stimuli, feelings of cold and being off balance, increased nausea, and limited social interactions to those of special importance.
- *Exhaustion* is characterized by confusion, emotional numbness, sudden loss of energy without exertion, difficulty sleeping or staying awake, inability to control body processes, and complete social withdrawal (Olson, 2007).

The experience of fatigue in cancer survivors is often multifactorial, and may be related to a symptom cluster (Wagner & Cella, 2004). It may be experienced with symptoms such as pain and sleep disturbances or may accompany depression. The National Comprehensive Cancer Network (NCCN) recommends screening for treatable etiologic causes for fatigue. These conditions may include anemia, side effects of medications, hypothyroidism, pulmonary dysfunction, sleep disturbance, fluid and electrolyte imbalances, adrenal insufficiency, cardiomyopathy, and emotional distress (NCCN, 2009). Radiation therapy may also cause prolonged fatigue after the completion of treatment.

Because fatigue is a subjective symptom it should be evaluated by self-reports. The NCCN Guidelines (2009) recommend screening patients with cancer at the initial visit and every subsequent visit, including during survivorship. The prompt may be a question such as, "How would you rate your fatigue over the last 7 days?" using a 0 to 10 scale (0 = no fatigue, 10 = worst fatigue you can imagine). Scores of 4 or greater indicate the need for further assessment for treatable conditions. Assessment should include a focused history regarding the cancer and treatment, medications, fatigue history, and physical assessment. Fatigue from medications such as opiates, antihistamines (e.g., diphenhydramine), and antiemetics (e.g., prochlorperazine) or from drug–drug interactions should be considered and managed appropriately (Mitchell *et al.*, 2007).

Interventions

According to the Oncology Nursing Society's (ONS) Putting Evidence into Practice Team® (PEP) for Fatigue, there are many studies investigating interventions for cancer-related fatigue, some providing sufficient evidence from studies or expert opinion to recommend them for clinical practice (ONS, 2009). The intervention for fatigue with the highest level of evidence was exercise in various forms (walking, cycling, swimming, resistive exercise), frequency, intensity, degree of supervision, and duration (Mitchell *et al.*, 2007). Referral of survivors to physical therapy and rehabilitation services may be useful in initiating exercise programs and rebuilding stamina.

Other interventions that the PEP team found likely to be effective included:

- Energy conservation and management
- Measures to optimize sleep quality
- Provision of education or information
- Relaxation
- Massage and healing touch

Surprisingly, the PEP review of the literature (2007) revealed there was benefit balanced with harms to managing anemia in people with cancer with hemoglobin <10 g/dl, but insufficient evidence to recommend it for clinical practice.

The NCCN Guidelines recommend patient and family education as the first line of treatment if other etiologic factors have been explored and eliminated. First, the survivor and family should be reassured that fatigue is not necessarily because of disease recurrence and progression, if this is indeed true. The general recommendations for managing fatigue from the NCCN (2009) include self-monitoring of fatigue levels, energy conservation measures, and the use of distraction (Table 4-4). Specific energy conservation and activity management strategies have been shown to have a statistically significant effect on fatigue measures (Barsevick *et al.*, 2004).

TABLE 4-4   Energy Conservation and Activity Management

Strategies	Rationale
Set priorities	Postpone low-priority activities
Pace activities	Balance activity and rest
Delegate responsibilities	Decrease responsibilities and allow others to help
Schedule activities at times of peak energy	Time activities to peak energy levels
Use labor-saving devices	Decrease energy exertion
Postpone nonessential activities	Allow for less energy exertion and more rest
Limit daytime naps to 20–30 minutes	Improve the quality of nighttime sleep
Structure the daily routine	Planned schedule facilitates regular exertion and times of more energy
Attend to one activity at a time	Stay focused and minimize burden of other responsibilities

Source: NCCN, v.1.2009

Additionally, other nonpharmacologic interventions may be useful in dealing with the experience of fatigue. Progressive muscle relaxation, yoga, healing touch, and massage may all improve sleep and decrease the experience of fatigue and other QOL indicators (ONS, 2009). Educational interventions to teach survivors and families about energy conservation and activity management may be useful in planning daily activities. Psychosocial interventions such as cognitive behavioral therapy, attention-restoring therapy, nutritional consultation, and strategies to enhance sleep quality are also recommended in the NCCN Guidelines.

Pharmacologic interventions may be useful for fatigue by improving energy levels, decreasing anxiety and depression, and improving the quality of sleep. Also, the treatment of anemia with human erythropoietin has shown some improvement in fatigue and increased vigor for those patients with Hgb <10 g/dl with a target of Hgb level of 11–12 g/dl (Bohlius *et al.*, 2004; Cella, Dobrez, & Glaspy, 2003).

Classes of drugs that may be useful in treating fatigue include psychostimulants (e.g., methylphenidate and modafinil), antidepressants (e.g., paroxetine and bupropion), and sleep medication (e.g., zolpidem). The use of paroxetine to treat fatigue has produced mixed findings in several studies, although it has been shown to improve depression. In a small study, bupropion improved fatigue in 13 of 15 patients with various cancer diagnoses (Cullum, Wojciechowski, Pelletier, & Simpson, 2004). Because most of the studies have explored fatigue in patients undergoing treatment, ongoing studies are needed to determine the effectiveness of specific medications for the experience of fatigue in cancer survivors.

Summary

The experience of fatigue has significant implications for the physical and psychosocial functioning of cancer survivors. Fatigue is often multifactorial and may be caused by physiologic conditions as well as overlap with other symptoms, such as pain and depression. Numerous nonpharmacologic and pharmacologic interventions have been studied to help survivors and their families deal with fatigue. Exercise and psychoeducational interventions appear to have the most significant effects on fatigue levels, but other interventions such as progressive relaxation and massage may also improve energy levels. Oncology nurses can assess fatigue at every visit with survivors and provide education and support to improve energy and offer referrals for more intensive evaluation and interventions.

References

Barsevick, A. M., Dudley, W., Beck, S., Sweeney, C., Whitmer, K., & Nail, L. (2004). A randomized clinical trial of energy conservation for patients with cancer-related fatigue. *Cancer, 100,* 1302–1310.

Bohlius, J., Langensiepen, S., Schwarzer, G., Seidenfeld, J., Piper, M., Bennet, C., et al. (2004). Erythropoietin for patients with malignant disease. *Cochrane Database of Systematic Reviews, 3,* CD003407.

Cella, D., Dobrez, D., & Glaspy, J. (2003). Control of cancer-related anemia with erythropoietic agents: A review of evidence for improved quality of life and clinical outcomes. *Annals of Oncology, 14,* 511–519.

Cullum, J. L., Wojciechowski, A. E., Pelletier, G., & Simpson, J. S. (2004). Bupropion sustained release treatment reduces fatigue in cancer patients. *Canadian Journal of Psychiatry, 49,* 139–144

Mitchell, S. A., Beck, S. L., Hood, L. E., Moore, K., & Tanner, E. R. (2007). Putting Evidence into Practice: Evidence-based interventions for fatigue during and following cancer and its treatment. *Clinical Journal of Oncology Nursing, 11*(1), 99–113.

Mock, V. (2004). Evidence-based treatment for cancer-related fatigue. *Journal of the National Cancer Institute Monographs, 32,* 112–118.

Nail, L. M. (2002). Fatigue in patients with cancer. *Oncology Nursing Forum, 29,* 537.

Nail, L. M. (2004). My get up and go got up and went: Fatigue in people with cancer. *Journal of the National Cancer Institute Monographs, 32,* 72–75.

National Comprehensive Cancer Network. (2009). NCCN Clinical Practice Guidelines in Oncology: Cancer-related Fatigue. Retrieved February 11, 2009, from www.nccn.org/professionals/physician_gls/PDF/fatigue.pdf

Olson, K. (2007). A new way of thinking about fatigue: A reconceptualization. *Oncology Nursing Forum, 34,* 93–99.

Oncology Nursing Society. (2009) Outcomes Resource Area. Putting Evidence into Practice: Fatigue. Retrieved February 11, 2009, from http://www.ons.org/outcomes/volume1/fatigue.shtml

Wagner, L. I., & Cella, D. (2004). Fatigue and cancer: Causes, prevalence and treatment approaches. *British Journal of Cancer, 91,* 822–828.

Bibliography

Mock, V. (2003). Clinical excellence through evidence-based practice: Fatigue management as a model. *Oncology Nursing Forum, 30,* 787–796.

Morrow, G. R., Shelke, A. R., Roscoe, J. A., Hickok, J. T., & Mustian, K. (2005). Management of cancer-related fatigue. *Cancer Investigation, 23,* 229–239.

Sarhill, N., Walsh, D., Nelson, K. A., Willey, J., Shen, L., Palmer, J. L., *et al.* (2001). Methylphenidate for fatigue in advanced cancer: A prospective open-label pilot study. *American Journal of Hospice and Palliative Care, 18,* 187–192.

PERIPHERAL NEUROPATHY

Ellen M. Lavoie Smith

Introduction

Chemotherapy-induced peripheral neuropathy (CIPN) occurs frequently in cancer survivors. It is caused when peripheral sensory, motor, and autonomic nerves become damaged by neurotoxic chemotherapeutic agents. This section begins by describing CIPN risk factors, signs, symptoms, and adverse outcomes. Emphasis is placed on prospective nurse assessment of neuropathy signs and symptoms. This section concludes with a brief review of known prevention and treatment strategies with a focus on what nurses can do to minimize CIPN-related problems.

Risk Factors

Only certain types of chemotherapeutic drugs cause peripheral neuropathy. These drugs are listed in Table 4-5. In addition, large single and cumulative dosages, prolonged infusion times, increased dose intensity (less time between treatments), and administration of multiple neurotoxic agents are factors that can increase CIPN risk (Hausheer, Schilsky, Bain, Berghorn, & Lieberman, 2006; Ocean & Vahdat, 2004; Quasthoff & Hartung, 2002; Verstappen, Heimans, Hoekman, & Postma, 2003).

In addition to neurotoxic chemotherapeutic drugs, several comorbid conditions can cause peripheral neuropathy, such as diabetes, peripheral vascular disease, HIV infection, B vitamin deficiency, alcoholism, and degenerative neurologic disorders such as Charcot-Marie-Tooth disease (Hausheer *et al.*, 2006; Ocean & Vahdat, 2004;

TABLE 4-5 Chemotherapeutic Drugs Causing Peripheral Neuropathy

Ara-C*	Gemcitabine*	Paclitaxel
Bortezomib	Hexamethylmelamine	Suramin[†]
Carboplatin	Ifosfamide*	Thalidomide
Cisplatin	Interferon-α*	Vinblastine
Docetaxel	Misonidazole	Vincristine
Ixabepalone[†]	Oxaliplatin	Vindesine[†]
Etoposide*	Procarbazine	Vinorelbine

*Rarely causes CIPN.
[†]Investigational.
Reprinted from Diagnosis, Management, and Evaluation of Chemotherapy - Induced Peripheral Neuropathy. Frederick H. Hausheer, Richard L. Schilsky, Stacey Bain, Elmer J. Berghorn and Frank Lieberman (2006) with permission from Elsevier.

Quasthoff & Hartung, 2002; Verstappen *et al.*, 2003; Visovsky, Meyer, Roller, & Poppas, 2008; Windebank & Grisold, 2008). CIPN signs and symptoms may be more severe and protracted when neurotoxic agents are administered to individuals with these comorbid conditions (Hausheer *et al.*, 2006; Visovsky *et al.*, 2008). Therefore, it is important to assess for the presence of comorbid risk factors before chemotherapeutic agents are prescribed, because anticancer treatment with nonneurotoxic alternatives may be indicated.

Lastly, there is emerging evidence suggesting that there are genetic-based variations in the body's ability to metabolize neurotoxic drugs (McWhinney, Goldberg, & McLeod, 2009; Mielke, 2007). These genetic variations may account for unexplained differences in CIPN when comparing neurotoxicity among cancer survivors with otherwise similar clinical risk factors. For the future, pharmacogenetic research will help us to identify these high-risk patients via genetic testing performed on blood, urine, or saliva. Genetic testing results will guide treatment choices so that those determined to be at high risk for developing CIPN will be identified in advance and alternative treatments can be chosen.

❀ Signs and Symptoms

Chemotherapy induced peripheral neuropathy signs and symptoms fall into three main categories: sensory, motor, and autonomic. Sensory signs and symptoms occur most frequently and typically develop over time after repeated administration of neurotoxic chemotherapeutic agents. In some cases, symptoms worsen for months after chemotherapy treatments have ended and pose significant problems for cancer survivors. Common sensory symptoms include bilateral numbness, tingling, and/or burning sensations experienced mainly in the feet and hands. These uncomfortable sensations may become more than just annoying, and may be described as actually painful. Sensory signs and symptoms typically begin in the toes and progress proximally as neuropathy becomes more severe. This occurs because the tips of the longest nerves are damaged first. Therefore, a patient with symptoms extending above the ankles has more severe neuropathy than a patient with symptoms only in the toes. Fingertip and hand signs and symptoms usually occur once lower extremity symptoms have progressed above the ankle. Therefore, CIPN in both upper and lower extremities is indicative of more severe neuropathy. Lastly, one neurotoxic chemotherapeutic agent, oxaliplatin, causes an unusual but transient cold-induced numbness and tingling occurring in the hands, feet, and oropharynx when exposed to cold temperatures (e.g., drinking cold drinks, touching cold objects, cold weather).

Muscle weakness also can occur when peripheral nerves are damaged. Weakness occurs most often in cancer survivors receiving high M^2 and/or high cumulative dosages of neurotoxic agents. Moreover, certain neurotoxic drugs are more likely to lead to motor weakness than others. For example, significant motor weakness is reported to occur more often in cancer survivors receiving vinca alkaloids, suramin, and bortezomib than in those receiving other neurotoxic agents (Hausheer *et al.*, 2006; Windebank & Grisold, 2008).

Constipation and orthostatic hypotension are the most common indicators of autonomic CIPN; however, impotence and urinary retention also can occur. Caused mainly by the vinca alkaloids, constipation occurs when autonomic nerves controlling gastrointestinal motility become impaired. In severe cases, constipation can progress to paralytic ileus or megacolon (Low, Vernino, & Suarez, 2003). Symptoms of orthostatic hypotension such as tachycardia and dizziness when standing occur because of the autonomic nervous system's inability to trigger lower-extremity venous constriction in response to sudden position changes.

Although occurring less frequently, neurotoxic chemotherapeutic agents also can damage cranial nerves. For example, vincristine-related jaw pain and hoarseness are symptoms of cranial nerve neuropathy (Windebank & Grisold, 2008).

❦ Adverse Outcomes

Chemotherapy-induced peripheral neuropathy can lead to many negative outcomes for cancer survivors. For example, many cancer survivors experience extremely uncomfortable and even painful neuropathy that is difficult to control. Pain as well as weakness in the hands and feet may limit the cancer survivor's ability to perform everyday activities. Survivors may have difficulty walking because of pain, weakness, altered balance, or frequent tripping, placing them at increased risk of falling. It may become difficult for cancer survivors to dress, hold objects, write, or participate in hobbies. Moreover, driving ability can become compromised because of decreased sensation and motor function in the feet and ankles.

Another very significant negative outcome of CIPN is that severe symptoms can necessitate dose reductions of lifesaving chemotherapeutic medications. In turn, these dose reductions may compromise the cancer survivor's chance for long-term cancer control and cure. For some, these negative consequences are short lived, as symptoms resolve over 6 to 12 months. However, for others, CIPN may take several years to improve or never completely resolve, resulting in long-term disability and suffering.

Assessment

One challenge to date has been the lack of attention to CIPN assessment. CIPN is a difficult symptom for many cancer survivors to describe. Therefore, many do not report their symptoms because of an inability to describe what they are feeling. In addition, cancer survivors may hesitate to tell their healthcare team about CIPN out of concern that they will no longer be able to receive treatments perceived to be critical to their survival. In addition to patient factors, healthcare professionals historically have not paid adequate attention to subjective and objective CIPN measurement because of the lack of easy-to-use, reliable, and valid measurement approaches (Smith, Beck, & Cohen, 2008). However, there are several simple assessment approaches that nurses can use to prospectively monitor CIPN. First, all cancer survivors should undergo a baseline symptom assessment. Keeping in mind that worse neuropathy equates to more proximal symptoms, nurses should ask cancer survivors to describe *where* they feel symptoms; that is, how far do numbness, tingling, and/or pain extend proximally from the toes. In addition, cancer survivors should be assessed for the presence of symptoms in the hands *and* feet with recognition that both upper and lower extremity symptoms indicate more advanced CIPN. Nurses should assess for frequent tripping or falls either because of motor weakness, foot drop, impaired balance, or orthostatic symptoms. For cancer survivors receiving vinca alkaloids, nurses should assess for constipation, jaw pain, and hoarseness.

Nurses also should assess for CIPN-related changes in functional status, as well as psychological and psychosocial outcomes. For example, the cancer survivor employed as a grocery store cashier may no longer be able to remain on their feet for prolonged time periods because of CIPN-related pain, thereby compromising their ability to meet the usual job requirements. In turn, the cancer survivor may be faced with economic ramifications because of unemployment or disability, as well as an associated detrimental effect on mood and QOL.

In addition to subjective symptom assessment, a physical examination focused on CIPN signs should be performed prior to each chemotherapy treatment. Nurses should learn to perform and interpret a simple yet comprehensive CIPN physical exam that includes assessment of tendon reflexes, strength, pinprick or temperature sensation, and vibratory sensation. Although a comprehensive description of how to perform and interpret a CIPN-focused exam is beyond the scope of this section, a few important tips are outlined in the following.

Similar to subjective symptoms, proximal reflex loss is associated with more severe neuropathy. Therefore, check the Achilles reflexes (the most distal reflex) first. If the Achilles reflexes are normal, the remaining more proximal reflexes also should be normal. If *only* the Achilles reflexes are abnormal (diminished or absent), this suggests less severe CIPN than if the Achilles' *and* patellar reflexes (the next proximal reflex) were abnormal. Ultimately, most cancer survivors receiving neurotoxic agents lose all reflexes. Although not problematic for patients, loss of tendon reflexes is an important early sign that should not be overlooked, because tendon reflex loss will most likely precede other CIPN signs and symptoms.

In addition to reflexes, nurses should assess the patient's strength in the toes, ankles, legs, fingers, wrists, and arms. Assessing the patient's ability to feel sharpness and vibration also is important. To make these assessments, first ask the patient to close his or her eyes. Then, touch a sharp object to the toes, such as the edge of a broken wooden tongue depressor. Ask the patient to describe what he or she feels. Allow the patient to choose descriptive sentences, such as, "It feels like a pencil point" or "It feels sharp." If the patient does not feel sharpness, repeatedly touch the object to the skin in an ascending fashion, moving up the foot to the ankle, calves, knees, and so on. Ask the patient to tell you what he or she feels all along the way. By doing so, the nurse should be able to determine at what point the sensation becomes normal again. The nurse can use the same approach to assess vibratory sensation by applying a vibrating 128 Hz tuning fork to the bony surface of the patient's great toe (or index finger). The nurse places his or her finger under the patient's toe or finger. The nurse should feel the vibration *through* the patient's toe or finger for at least as long as the patient feels it. If the patient is unable to feel the "buzzing" sensation, or feels it for less time than the nurse, vibratory sensation is impaired. If vibration sensation is normal in the toes, there is no need to proceed proximally. However, if vibration sensibility is impaired, the nurse should repeat the assessments proximally, next assessing the patient's ability to feel the buzzing at the malleolus, then at the anterior lower leg, knee, fingers, and so on. The level of normal sensation is an indicator of neuropathy proximal extension. Pinprick and vibratory sensation testing should be assessed in the upper extremities if lower-extremity sensation is impaired. Temperature sensation can be substituted for pinprick sensation (preferable in children) and is assessed by touching the cold tuning fork to the patient's skin in an ascending fashion, starting at the toes. The patient is prompted to describe what is felt. If normal temperature sensation is present, the patient will state that the tuning fork feels cold or cool.

Results for subjective and objective measurement can be scored using a variety of composite instruments such as the Total Neuropathy Score (Smith *et al.*, 2008). In addition, several other assessment instruments have been developed that assess CIPN-related changes in functional status and QOL. These instruments include the FACT-GOG/Ntx (Calhoun *et al.*, 2003), the FACT-Taxane (Cella, Peterman, Hudgens, Webster, & Socinski, 2003), the Ntx-12 (Kopec *et al.*, 2006), and the QLQ-CIPN20 (Postma *et al.*, 2005). Neuropathy grading scales also can be used such as the National Cancer Institute Common Terminology Criteria (NCI-CTC), but these scales have been criticized for having floor effects and suboptimal sensitivity (Postma *et al.*, 1998). Therefore, the main problem is that many neuropathy measurement approaches have not undergone rigorous scientific testing to assure that the instruments are reliable and valid. Research is ongoing in this area.

⊗ Prevention and Treatment

Several CIPN prevention and treatment pharmacologic agents have been evaluated. These agents include intravenous calcium and magnesium, vitamin E, glutamine, glutathione, N-acetylcysteine, acetyl-L-carnitine, xaliproden, tricyclic antidepressants, anticonvulsants, alpha lipoic acid, and human leukemia factor (Amara, 2008; Visovsky, Collins, Abbott, Aschenbrenner, & Hart, 2007; Wolf, Barton,

Kottschade, Grothey, & Loprinzi, 2008). Unfortunately, despite ongoing research in this area, there is insufficient evidence to justify routine use of these agents (Visovsky *et al.*, 2007; Wolf *et al.*, 2008). Vitamin E, calcium/magnesium, glutamine, glutathione, N-acetylcysteine, oxcarbazepine, and xaliproden hold the most promise to date. However, these agents must undergo further testing via large, randomized trials before determining their true efficacy.

Moreover, there is insufficient evidence justifying nonpharmacologic interventions for CIPN (Visovsky *et al.*, 2007). Future research conducted in cancer survivors is needed to test the efficacy of approaches such as acupuncture, physical therapy targeting strength and balance, occupational therapy, exercise, and educational interventions.

Although there are no known agents that will prevent or treat CIPN-related nerve injury, there are several medications that may be effective in decreasing pain from CIPN. These medications include gabapentin, pregabalin, duloxetine, tramadol, and methadone. Other antidepressants, anticonvulsants, and opioids also may be effective. However, trial and error may be needed before discovering the most efficacious, well-tolerated drug or combination of drugs, and referral to an expert in the treatment of neuropathic pain is recommended. Research in this area also is ongoing.

❀ The Nurse's Role

Nurses can play a major role in minimizing CIPN-related problems. First, nurses are in a perfect position to assess cancer survivors for CIPN signs and symptoms, because cancer survivors often share stories about how CIPN is affecting their lives while interacting with nurses during chemotherapy infusions, over the telephone during routine triage calls, or while receiving daily inpatient and outpatient nursing care. Because

CIPN is rarely life threatening, cancer survivors often seem reluctant to share these stories with their physician out of concern for wasting the physician's time with what the patient believes the physician will judge to be unimportant. However, when given an opportunity to share their concerns, cancer survivors are truly grateful for focused attention on the problem. More specifically, attention to careful CIPN assessment, treatment of painful symptoms, and patient education can be effective strategies that improve patient function and QOL.

Regarding educational interventions, there is a significant amount of CIPN-related information that should be shared with cancer survivors. Table 4-6 provides a summary of important CIPN-related educational topics. Cancer survivors appreciate learning about CIPN causes and the expected recovery timeline. Survivors should be taught to report CIPN signs and symptoms, particularly when receiving ongoing neurotoxic chemotherapy. Emphasis should be placed on the importance of balancing chemotherapy treatment toxicity with efficacy and that neglecting to report CIPN could lead to irreversible discomfort and functional disability. Let the patient know that, in many cases, chemotherapy dose reductions or alternative chemotherapy agent substitu-

---

TABLE 4-6   Chemotherapy-Induced Peripheral Neuropathy-Related Cancer Survivor-Focused Educational Topics

1. Common Causes and Clinical Course
2. Reporting CIPN Signs and Symptoms
3. Safety
4. Managing Symptoms of Autonomic Neuropathy
5. Treatment Strategies for CIPN-related Neuropathic Pain

tions will not significantly compromise cancer treatment effectiveness. Also explain that you and/or the physician will be closely monitoring for changes in CIPN signs and symptoms so that problems can be addressed early. It is also important to teach the patient about safety factors. Cancer survivors should wear hard-soled footwear, avoid exposing their hands and feet to extreme temperatures, and remove items such as throw rugs or other clutter that could lead to trips and falls. For those with impaired balance, instruct the patient to always turn the lights on if getting up at night. This is important because when there is diminished foot sensation, the cancer survivor must use visual clues to monitor where his or her feet are in space in order to avoid losing balance. Walking with a broad-based gait is another strategy that aids impaired balance. Strategies to minimize orthostatic hypotension such as slow position changes should be emphasized, as should constipation management strategies. Lastly, cancer survivors should know that there are medications that can be used to treat CIPN-related pain, which, if effective, can improve sleep, daily function, and overall mood.

☮ Summary

Chemotherapy-induced peripheral neuropathy can be an extremely challenging long-term outcome of cancer treatment for many cancer survivors. Although much is still unknown regarding how to best prevent and treat CIPN, nurses can make a tremendous positive impact on cancer survivors' function and QOL through increased attention to proactive assessment, treatment of CIPN-related pain, and educational/support interventions. In addition, increased attention is now being placed on discovering better ways to predict, monitor, prevent, and treat CIPN. Therefore, cancer survivors can be more hopeful than ever that help is on the way.

References

Amara, S. (2008). Oral glutamine for the prevention of chemotherapy-induced peripheral neuropathy. *The Annals of Pharmacotherapy, 42*, 1481–1485.

Calhoun, E. A., Welshman, E. E., Chang, C. H., Lurain, J. R., Fishman, D. A., Hunt, T. L., *et al.* (2003). Psychometric evaluation of the Functional Assessment Of Cancer Therapy/Gynecologic Oncology Group-neurotoxicity (Fact/GOG-ntx) questionnaire for patients receiving systemic chemotherapy. *International Journal of Gynecological Cancer, 13*(6), 741–748.

Cella, D., Peterman, A., Hudgens, S., Webster, K., & Socinski, M. A. (2003). Measuring the side effects of taxane therapy in oncology: The functional assessment of cancer therapy-taxane (FACT-taxane). *Cancer, 98*(4), 822–831.

Hausheer, F. H., Schilsky, R. L., Bain, S., Berghorn, E. J., & Lieberman, F. (2006). Diagnosis, management, and evaluation of chemotherapy-induced peripheral neuropathy. *Seminars in Oncology, 33*(1), 15–49.

Kopec, J. A., Land, S. R., Cecchini, R. S., Ganz, P. A., Cella, D., Costantino, J. P., *et al.* (2006). Validation of a self-reported neurotoxicity scale in patients with operable colon cancer receiving oxaliplatin. *Supportive Oncology, 4*(8), W1–W7.

Low, P.A., Vernino, S., & Suarez, G. (2003). Autonomic dysfunction in peripheral nerve disease. *Muscle & Nerve, 27*(6), 646–661.

McWhinney, S. R., Goldberg, R. M., & McLeod, H. L. (2009). Platinum neurotoxicity pharmacogenetics. *Molecular Cancer Therapeutics, 8*(1), 10–16.

Mielke, S. (2007). Individualized pharmacotherapy with paclitaxel. *Current Opinion in Oncology, 19*(6), 586–589.

Ocean, A. J., & Vahdat, L. T. (2004). Chemotherapy-induced peripheral neuropathy: Pathogenesis and emerging therapies. *Supportive Care in Cancer, 12*(9), 619–625.

Postma, T. J., Aaronson, N. K., Heimans, J. J., Muller, M. J., Hildebrand, J. G., Delattre, J.Y., *et al.* (2005). The development of an EORTC quality of life questionnaire to assess chemotherapy-induced peripheral neuropathy: The QLQ-CIPN20. *European Journal of Cancer, 41*(8), 1135–1139.

Postma, T. J., Heimans, J. J., Muller, M. J., Ossenkoppele, G. J., Vermorken, J. B., & Aaronson, N. K. (1998). Pitfalls in grading severity of chemotherapy-induced peripheral neuropathy. *Annals of Oncology, 9*(7), 739–744.

Quasthoff, S., & Hartung, H. P. (2002). Chemotherapy-induced peripheral neuropathy. *Journal of Neurology, 249*(1), 9–17.

Smith, E. L., Beck, S. L., & Cohen, J. (2008). The total neuropathy score (TNS): A tool for measuring chemotherapy-induced peripheral neuropathy. *The Oncology Nursing Forum, 35*(102), 96–102.

Verstappen, C. C., Heimans, J. J., Hoekman, K., & Postma, T. J. (2003). Neurotoxic complications of chemotherapy in patients with cancer: Clinical signs and optimal management. *Drugs, 63*(15), 1549–1563.

Visovsky, C., Collins, M., Abbott, L., Aschenbrenner, J., & Hart, H. (2007). Putting evidence into practice: Evidence-based interventions for chemotherapy-induced peripheral neuropathy. *Clinical Journal of Oncology Nursing, 11*(6), 901–913.

Visovsky, C., Meyer, R. R., Roller, J., & Poppas, M. (2008). Evaluation and management of peripheral neuropathy in diabetic patients with cancer. *Clinical Journal of Oncology Nursing, 12*(2), 243–247.

Windebank, A. J., & Grisold, W. (2008). Chemotherapy-induced neuropathy. *Journal of the Peripheral Nervous System, 13*, 27–46.

Wolf, S., Barton, D., Kottschade, L., Grothey, A., & Loprinzi, C. (2008). Chemotherapy-induced peripheral neuropathy: Prevention and treatment strategies. *European Journal of Cancer, 44*(11), 1507–1515.

ANXIETY

Lisa Kennedy Sheldon

Introduction

A diagnosis of cancer can create anxiety and distress for patients and survivors. Even the prospect of finishing treatment creates fear of the future and uncertainty of recurrence. Nurses are ideally situated to assess cancer survivors for signs and symptoms of anxiety because of the extended periods of time they spend with patients. Anxiety may occur at different times over the trajectory of cancer survivorship as well as at the time of diagnosis. It may also be part of a preexisting anxiety disorder.

Feelings of anxiety may resurface during survivorship if hopes and expectations are challenged. During specific times, such as follow-up examinations and diagnostic testing, cancer survivors may reexperience distressing feelings and anxiety. For example, the revelation of metastatic disease or disease progression, increasing symptoms such as pain, or the prospect of ending active treatment may stimulate anxiety and fear again. Further assessment may be needed to determine the person's experience and the need for further evaluation and/or intervention. When nurses provide acknowledgment of their distress by carefully exploring their concerns, they provide support that may be a therapeutic intervention.

Some people may have preexisting anxiety or a generalized anxiety disorder that creates increasing worry after a cancer diagnosis (Derogatis *et al.*, 1983). A generalized anxiety disorder is defined as chronic, uncontrollable nervousness, fearfulness, and a sense of worry (Lantz, 2002). People with a generalized anxiety disorder may have received treatment previously for their anxiety, including counseling and/or medications. Determination of an underlying condition, previous treatment strategies for the disorder, and current anxiety levels helps direct further interventions during cancer survivorship.

⑧ Signs and Symptoms

Symptoms of anxiety include both psychological and physical manifestations. Feeling anxious is precipitated by stimulation of a general adaptation to stress, including both the sympathetic and autonomic nervous systems. High anxiety often precipitates physical symptoms related to activation of the autonomic nervous system (ANS) (Camp-Sorrell & Hawkins, 2000). Stimulation of the ANS may produce sweating, tachycardia, cold and clammy hands, dizziness, and diarrhea. Physical symptoms in the musculoskeletal system include trembling, shakiness and jumpiness, inability to relax, and restlessness.

Common physical symptoms of anxiety are:

- Tachycardia or palpitations
- Sweating
- Perception of dyspnea or shortness of breath
- Loss of appetite
- Headaches
- Restlessness or fidgeting
- Abdominal distress

Medical conditions and certain drugs may also cause anxiety. Hormone-secreting tumors, some medications, withdrawal from alcohol and drugs, or other physical symptoms such as pain may produce feelings of anxiety. It is important to assess other physical problems that may be causing the feelings of anxiety. Medical conditions that may cause anxiety include hormone-producing tumors such as pheochromocytoma, hypoxia and pulmonary embolism, congestive heart failure, hyperthyroidism, carcinoid syndrome, electrolyte imbalances, and the use of steroids and/or stimulants.

Anxiety, depression, and distress are often clustered when describing the experience of people with cancer. The term *distress* is often used instead of *anxiety* because it has less social stigma attached to it and may be easier for patients to discuss (NCCN, 2008). The actual incidence of anxiety has often been combined with depression in studies that evaluate psychiatric disorders in oncology patients. According to the landmark study by the Psychosocial Collaborative Oncology Group, 47% of cancer patients had psychiatric disorders, 68% of whom had reactive or situational anxiety and depression (Derogatis, Morrow, & Fettig, 1983). Further examination revealed that 90% of these disorders were reactions to the cancer or manifestations of the cancer itself. Unfortunately, <10% of people with cancer and anxiety were identified as needing psychosocial interventions.

🎗 Assessment

Whenever it occurs across the cancer spectrum, anxiety is one manifestation of emotional distress. The National Comprehensive Cancer Network (NCCN) has included the management of anxiety within their guidelines for the management of distress in cancer patients (NCCN, 2008). According to the NCCN guidelines, distress is perceived as occurring along a continuum from normal feelings of sadness and vulnerability to problems that may become disabling, such as anxiety. Using the VAS (NCCN, 2008), people can rate their distress on a scale of 0 to 10 (0 = no distress, 10 = worst distress of their life). Scores of 4 or higher on the VAS indicate the need further evaluation using the subcscale for specific concerns that are causing distress as well as further assessment by the nurse (NCCN, 2008) (Table 4-7).

If symptoms of anxiety persist and/or increase, patients may need further evaluation and interventions. Patients should be reassessed

TABLE 4-7   Periods of Increased Vulnerability to Anxiety

Finding a suspicious symptom

During workup

At the time of diagnosis

Awaiting treatment

During arduous treatment cycles

Change in treatment modality

End of treatment and survivorship issues

Discharge from hospital

Before medical follow-up visits and surveillance

Minor symptoms that could represent recurrence of disease

Treatment failure with recurrence and/or progression

Advanced cancer or worsening symptoms

Transition to hospice/palliative care

Awareness of the end of life

Adapted from: Camp-Sorrell & Hawkins, 2000; NCCN, 2005; Sheldon, 2008.

every 3 weeks to assess their response to the medications. Depressive symptoms may be seen in association with anxiety in some patients. If a patient is suicidal, he or she should immediately be referred to a mental healthcare provider at a center or hospital. The following guidelines may indicate the need for referral to a mental health professional, social worker, and/or pastoral counselor:

- Score ≥4 on the VAS (NCCN, 2005)
- Excessive worries and fears
- Excessive sadness
- Unclear thinking

- Despair and hopelessness
- Severe family problems
- Spiritual crises
- Suicidal ideation

✺ Interventions

Psychosocial Interventions

Treating anxiety requires careful assessment to determine the source of the concerns. First, possible physical and medical causes of anxiety should be explored and then treated appropriately. After eliminating medical causes of anxiety, psychosocial and psychoeducational interventions are the mainstay of treatment for anxiety. Psychoeducational interventions are aimed at providing the necessary information if concerns exist about the unknown, or conclusions have been reached that are not based on factual information. Oncology nurses routinely help survivors understand information and address these concerns.

There are many different types of psychosocial interventions to diminish patient anxiety. Psychosocial interventions range from impromptu support to individual or group counseling, psychoeducational interventions, and even telephone-linked care. Psychosocial interventions such as cognitive behavior stress management (Antoni *et al.*, 2006) and cognitive existential therapy (Kissane *et al.*, 2003) have both been shown to decrease anxiety in people with cancer. Pastoral counseling may be necessary to address survivors' spiritual concerns.

Psychosocial and psychoeducational interventions may include:

- Individual therapy
- Group therapy and support groups
- Psychoeducational sessions
- Telephone-based interventions such as telephone interpersonal counseling (TIP-C)

- Spiritually based psychotherapy/pastoral counseling
- Hypnosis (self and guided).

Communication skills are not only part of assessing the responses of cancer survivors; they may also be therapeutic in themselves. Opening conversations that allow survivors to discuss their concerns, such as fears of recurrence or worries about unrelieved pain, may be helpful in decreasing anxiety (Stiles, Shuster, & Harrigan, 1992). Choosing the best responses to survivor concerns depends on the experience and training of the oncology nurse. Oncology nurses spend extended periods of time with people with cancer. They often hear their concerns and spontaneously provide support and information to help alleviate specific concerns.

Acknowledging the emotional impact of these concerns is an additive way to respond to them and may be therapeutic. The NURS pneumonic has been used to describe the steps of empathetic responsiveness in patient-centered interviewing (Smith, 2002). The following steps have been described to help nurses and other healthcare providers respond to patient emotional expressions such as anxiety and distress.

- N—Name the feeling. "I can see that you are really worried about this test."
- U—Understand the patient's experience. "Many patients feel concerned when waiting for test results."
- R—Respect the patient's coping. "You are doing the best you can to deal with this situation and help your family, too."
- S—Support the patient. "I would like to help you get through this time."

When nurses respond empathetically, survivors feel more comfortable disclosing their concerns in a nonjudgmental and respectful climate. By reflecting the emotional content and supporting the survivor's coping strategies, the nurse empowers the patient and yet also identifies anxiety that may require further intervention to support the patient's functioning. When the nurse establishes that routine psychosocial support is not alleviating the patient's anxiety, then further pharmacologic interventions and/or referral may be needed for the patient.

Psychosocial and psychoeducational interventions have been the subject of research and systematic reviews of the literature (Andrykowski & Manne, 2006). There is sufficient evidence to recommend psychosocial interventions to reduce levels of anxiety in cancer patients and psychoeducational interventions. Although it is difficult to identify which type of intervention benefits each survivor, it may be that the nurse should assess the individual, identifying strategies that have worked previously as one way to identify the best psychosocial interventions for the current situation. The establishment of a therapeutic nurse–patient relationship allows the nurse to tailor the type and amount of psychosocial and psychoeducational interventions to meet the needs of the individual.

Pharmacologic Interventions

When psychosocial and/or psychoeducational interventions are insufficient to treat the survivor's anxiety, pharmacologic treatments may be added to alleviate anxiety and distress. Pharmacologic agents should always be combined with psychosocial interventions. Medications may include anxiolytics (antianxiety), antidepressants, azapirones, antihistamines, and atypical neuroleptics.

Anxiolytic Medications

Anxiolytic (antianxiety) medications are used to decrease anxiety in people with situational anxiety and generalized anxiety disorders. Situational anxiety is described as anxiety in relation to specific causative events in their environment. This type of anxiety is usually self-limited but may cause acute anxiety. For example, anxiety preceding follow-up scans may be relieved by hearing the results.

On the other hand, generalized anxiety disorders are long-term disorders (>6 months) characterized by excessive worry and anxiety about numerous events (Camp-Sorrell & Hawkins, 2000). Although few studies have examined the effects of anxiolytics on cancer survivors, anxiolytics have been used and studied in many patient populations and are recommended by the NCCN guidelines (2005) as one pharmacologic treatment for anxiety. The anxiolytics that are most frequently used are benzodiazepines (lorazepam, diazepam), hydroxyzine, and buspirone (Table 4-8).

TABLE 4-8 Medications for the Treatment of Anxiety

Medication	Dosage	Side effects	Contraindications	PO/IV
Benzodiazepines				
Lorazepam Example: Ativan	0.5–2.0 mg Every 8–12 hours	CNS depression, sedation, dizziness, weakness, transient memory impairment, disorientation, sleep disturbances, agitation, and abuse potential	Acute narrow angle glaucoma Caution with opioids and other CNS depressants, including alcohol	PO/IV
Diazepam Example: Valium	2–10 mg 2–4 times daily Increase gradually	CNS depression, impaired coordination, fatigue, changes in libido/appetite	Acute narrow angle glaucoma Caution with substance/alcohol abuse, depression	PO/IV

(continued)

TABLE 4-8 (continued)

Medication	Dosage	Side effects	Contraindications	PO/IV
Alprazolam Example: Xanax	Start at 0.25–0.5 mg/tid May increase every 4 days to 4 mg/day in divided doses	CNS depression, fatigue, impaired coordination and memory, changes in libido and/or appetite	Open-angle glaucoma Use with caution in suicidal ideation Avoid abrupt cessation	PO
Clonazepam Example: Klonopin	0.5–1.5 mg/day	Nausea, drowsiness, impaired cognition, irritability, impaired coordination and balance	Elderly, those at risk for falls, schizophrenics Not recommended for those under 18 years	PO
Azapirones				
Buspirone Example: BuSpar	7.5 mg bid initially then may increase 5 mg/day every 2–3 days up to 60 mg/day	Dizziness, nausea headache, nervousness, dream disturbances, insomnia	Caution with other CNS drugs, renal and hepatic failure Do not use with concomitant MAOIs Do not take with grapefruit juice	PO

TABLE 4-8 (continued)

Antihistamines

Hydroxyzine Vistaril	25–50 mg every 4–6 hours	Drowsiness, dry mouth, tremor, convulsions	Caution in the elderly	PO/IV

Antidepressants

Paroxetine Example: Paxil	Start 20 mg/day and increase by 20 mg at 1 week intervals up to 60 mg/day	Asthenia, sweating, decreased appetite, dizziness, somnolence	Seizure disorder Cardiovascular disease Narrow-angle glaucoma	PO
Sertraline Example: Zoloft	Start 25–50 mg/day Increase at 1-week intervals	GI upset, insomnia, sexual dysfunction	Contraindicated in cardiovascular disease Monitor for mania/hypomania, hyperglycemia Use with caution in seizure disorders	PO
Escitalopram Example: Lexapro	10 mg, qd May increase to 20 mg qd	Nausea, insomnia, sexual dysfunction, fatigue	Do not use with concomitant MAOIs Avoid alcohol	PO
Venlafaxine Example: Effexor	75 mg/day May start at 37.5 mg/day for 4–7 days	GI upset, dizziness somnolence, insomnia, headache, sexual dysfunction	Caution with high blood pressure, heart disease, hypercholesterolemia, seizure disorders	PO

(continued)

TABLE 4-8 (continued)

Medication	Dosage	Side effects	Contraindications	PO/IV
Mirtazapine Example: Remeron	15 mg/day May increase q 7 days up to 45 mg/day	Visual hallucinations, increased appetite, nightmares, drowsiness, headache	Do not use with concomitant MAOIs Avoid alcohol Use with caution with benzodi- azepines	PO
Atypical Neuroleptics				
Olanzapine Example: Zyprexa	5–10 mg/day	Tardive dyskinesia, dizziness sedation insomnia, orthostatic hypotension, weight gain	Avoid in elderly with dementia Not for IV use	PO/IM
Risperidone Example: Risperdal	1–3 mg/day Start at 0.5 mg/day in elderly	Extrapyramidal symptoms, dizziness, somnolence, nausea	Caution in the elderly Increased risk of CVA and death Hyperglycemia	PO
Other				
Propofol Example: Diprivan	Titrated IV dosage for sedation and anesthesia	Airway obstruction, apnea, hypoventilation	Sedative hypnotic for anesthesia	IV

Adapted from: Sheldon, Swanson, Dolce, Marsh, & Summers, 2008.
Abbreviations: IM, intramuscular; PO, oral; PR, per rectum; SC, subcutaneous; SL, sublingual; T, topical.

Complementary Therapies

Complementary therapies are increasingly being used to reduce anxiety and improve QOL. Survivors often seek additional therapies to improve their QOL and some examples of complementary therapies include:

- Guided imagery
- Yoga
- Progressive relaxation/relaxation exercises
- Massage including body and foot massage and partner-delivered massage
- Reflexology
- Self-hypnotic relaxation
- Reiki
- Aromatherapy
- Virtual reality
- Art therapy
- Stress reducing medical devices for needle phobia
- Meditation
- Exercise

Outcomes for people experiencing anxiety depend on the specific sources of concern. Psychosocial and psychoeducational interventions may help to decrease anxiety levels in people with cancer (Sheldon *et al.,* 2008). By decreasing anxiety, patients will function better in their roles and make decisions more efficiently, without undue distress. Some outcomes of effective treatment of anxiety include:

- Decreased distress
- Improved QOL
- Better functioning in roles
- Increased adherence to cancer treatment and follow-up
- More open and trusting relationships with healthcare providers

§ Summary

Living as a cancer survivor is fraught with emotional times, from hope to moments of fear and anxiety. Oncology nurses can help survivors manage their anxiety by recognizing vulnerable points in the cancer trajectory, providing psychosocial and psychoeducational interventions, supporting effective coping skills, and referring those people with severe anxiety for intensive therapy and/or pharmacologic management. Because ongoing anxiety can affect QOL and performance in life roles, it is important that nurses assess for anxiety and support cancer survivors along their journey.

References

Andrykowski, M. A., & Manne, S. L. (2006). Are psychological interventions effective and accepted by cancer patients? I. Standards and levels of evidence. *Annals of Behavioral Medicine, 32*(2), 93–97.

Antoni, M. H., Wiberley, S. R., Lechner, S. C., Kazi, M. S., Sifre, T., Urcuyo, M. S., *et al.*, (2006). Reduction of cancer-specific thought intrusions and anxiety symptoms with a stress management intervention among women undergoing treatment for breast cancer. *American Journal of Psychiatry, 163*(10), 1791–1797.

Camp-Sorrell, D., & Hawkins, R.A. (2000). Anxiety in *Clinical manual for the oncology advanced practice nurse.* Pittsburgh: Oncology Nursing Press.

Derogatis, L. R., Morrow, G. R., Fetting, J., Penman, D., Piasetsky, S., Schmale, A. M., *et al.* (1983). The prevalence of psychiatric disorders among cancer patients. *Journal of the American Medical Association, 249,* 751–757.

National Comprehensive Cancer Network and American Cancer Society. (2005). Distress: treatment guidelines for patients, version II. Retrieved December 1, 2008, from http://www.nccn.org/professionals/physician_gls/PDF/distress.pdf

Kissane, D. W., Bloch, S., Smith, G. C., Miach, P., Clarke, D. M., Ikin, J., *et al.*, (2003). Cognitive-existential group psychotherapy for women with primary breast cancer: A randomised controlled trial. *Psycho-Oncology, 12,* 532–546.

Lantz, M. (2002). Generalized anxiety in anxious times; helping older adults cope. *Clinical Geriatrics, 10,* 36–38.

Sheldon, L. K. (2008). Anxiety and people with cancer. In C. Brown (Ed.), *A guide to oncology symptom management.* Pittsburgh, PA: Oncology Nursing Society.

Sheldon, L. K., Swanson, S., Dolce, A., Marsh, K., & Summers, J. (2008). Putting evidence into practice: Evidence-based interventions for anxiety. *Clinical Journal of Oncology Nursing, 12*(5), 789–797.

Smith, R. C. (2002). *Patient-centered interviewing: An evidence-based method.* Philadelphia: Lippincott Williams & Wilkins.

Stiles, W. B., Shuster, P. L., & Harrigan, J. A. (1992). Disclosure and anxiety: A test of the fever model. *Journal of Personality and Social Psychology, 63,* 980–988.

Bibliography

Fulcher, C.D., Badger, T., Gubter, A.K., Marrs, J.A. & Reese, J.M. (2008). Putting evidence into practice (PEP): Depression. *Clinical Journal of Oncology Nursing, 12*(1), 131–140.

🎗 DEPRESSION

Lisa Kennedy Sheldon

🎗 Introduction

The diagnosis of a potentially life-shortening disease such as cancer profoundly affects people and may cause fear, uncertainty, anxiety, and depression. Up to 70% of people with cancer may experience depression at some point during the course of their treatment and survivorship, with 25% meeting the criteria for a major depressive disorder (Derogatis *et al.,* 1983; Payne & Massie, 2002). Depression is estimated to have a prevalence of 15–50% in breast cancer patients (Zabora, Britzenhofeszoc, Curbow, Hooker, & Piantados, 2001). Depression may occur as a result of situational factors such as the diagnosis or may be part of an ongoing depressive disorder. According to the 2004 LIVESTRONG poll, 49% of survivors felt their non-medical needs, including psychosocial concerns, were not met by the healthcare system. Emotional distress, including depression, can affect cancer recovery, and QOL (Fulcher, Badger, Gunter, Marrs, & Reese, 2008). Oncology nurses are in a unique position to assess survivors for emotional concerns, including depression, over the course of their treatment and into survivorship. Early assessment and identification of signs of depression facilitates more rapid interventions including psychosocial support, referral for ongoing counseling, and/or pharmacologic interventions.

Living after a diagnosis of cancer brings a variety of emotional responses. Some emotions, such as shock and disbelief, are acute right after diagnosis. Later, people receiving cancer treatment are more concerned about managing the side effects of treatment and reaching completion of the prescribed therapy. Sometimes the hardest part of adjustment to life after a cancer diagnosis occurs during the first 6 months after the treatment has completed. People fortify themselves for chemotherapy, radiation therapy, and surgery. Once treatment is finished, there's an emotional release of all the tension and anxiety that was held back during treatment. They often feel depressed, anxious, and have trouble sleeping and may even feel more fatigued than during treatment. This phase is also a time of fear: fear of recurrence of the disease, a shortened life span, and perhaps fear of ongoing symptoms such as pain. Preparing patients for this response allows them to realize this is a common reaction and that they will adjust and grow into a "new normal," the life after cancer treatment.

❀ Assessment

Across the trajectory, the impact of a cancer diagnosis influences cancer survivors' ability to function in their usual roles in their families, at work, and within the community. How people respond to cancer diagnoses varies by their personality, concerns, support systems, and the circumstances of their disease and treatment. Some cancer survivors are at increased risk for depression. These patients require careful assessment at every visit and possibly ongoing supportive interventions from mental health specialists. According to a review of the literature on the NCI Web site (2009), people with cancer who are at increased risk for depression include:

- Depression at time of diagnosis
- History of depression, previous treatment for psychiatric problems, and/or suicide attempts
- History of alcoholism and/or drug abuse
- Family history of depression or suicide

- Pancreatic, head, and neck cancers
- Lack of family support
- Additional life stressors
- Being single and/or unmarried
- Poorly controlled pain
- Increased physical impairment
- Advanced stage of cancer (adapted from NCI Web site, 2009; Roth & Holland, 1995)

Oncology nurses often spend extended periods of time with cancer survivors during treatment, gaining an understanding of their needs and concerns, patterns of adaptation, and family roles. Sometimes patients are reluctant to discuss their emotional concerns; perhaps they fear being a burden to their families or healthcare providers, maybe expressing these concerns would make them appear less than stoic about their diagnosis and treatment, or maybe they accept their feelings of sadness as part of the cancer journey. They may have frequent thoughts laced with shame and guilt, such as, "I brought this on myself," "God is punishing me," or "I'm letting my family down." Nursing interventions can facilitate disclosure of these emotional concerns, and this facilitated disclosure may be therapeutic in relieving distress by acknowledging feelings of sadness and supporting the survivor's available resources. It also provides an opportunity to further assess the survivor's depressive thoughts, risk of suicide, and need for referral and treatment.

One important aspect of assessing for depression in cancer survivors is the well-known incidence of depressive symptoms as a result of biophysical changes. Feelings of sadness and depression can be caused by numerous factors, including physical changes from the cancer, other comorbid conditions, medications, and/or treatment. Possible medical causes of depressive symptoms in cancer patients include uncontrolled pain, metabolic abnormalities such as hypercalcemia and anemia, endocrine abnormalities such as hypothyroidism, medications such as steroids, and chemotherapy (procarbazine and cytokine therapy with interferon-alfa and interleukin-2). It is important to consider biophysical causes of depressive symptoms in cancer survivors when assessing emotional responses to the disease and treatment.

Depression is defined by the *Diagnostic and Statistical Manual of Mental Disorders,* 4th edition (*DSM-IV*), as the presence of depressed mood or loss of interest or pleasure in nearly all activities for a period of at least 2 weeks. Additional signs of depression listed in the *DSM-IV* are echoed in the definition outlined by the National Cancer Institute (2009) as signs and symptoms of depression in cancer patients. These include:

- A depressed mood for most of the day on most days
- Diminished pleasure or interest in most activities
- Significant change in appetite and sleep patterns
- Psychomotor agitation or slowing
- Fatigue
- Feelings of worthlessness and excessive, inappropriate guilt
- Poor concentration
- Recurrent thoughts of death or suicide

Measuring a cancer survivor's emotional responses, including depression, has been done by different specialties, including psychiatry, psychology, social work, medicine, and nursing. Measurement of mental health and depressive symptoms in general has often been done using tools borrowed from psychiatry and psychology with measures such as the Beck Depression Inventory (BDI) (Beck, 1972; Beck, Steer, & Garbin, 1988) and the Hospital Anxiety and Depression Scale (HADS) (Zigmond & Snaith, 1983). Sometimes emotional concerns have been considered part of assessing QOL or captured as the more global concept as "distress." Some of these measures, including paper and pencil tools and interviews, may be time consuming and unsuitable for quick and regular assessment during routine visits. Every healthcare setting that treats cancer survivors should find an efficient and reliable tool to assess for depression in cancer survivors to make it useful during routine visits.

Faster and simpler methods for assessing depressive signs and symptoms may be useful to oncology nurses and less of a burden to their patients. Examples include the "Two-Question Method," and the NCCN Distress Thermometer.

The Two-Question Method

1. "Are you depressed or do you feel depressed most of the time?"
2. If yes to number 1, "Is it difficult to find joy in the things that used to make you happy?"

If the survivor answers yes to both questions, he or she requires referral to another provider for more intensive assessment and possibly treatment.

The National Comprehensive Cancer Network Distress Thermometer

One way to assess for emotional concerns in general is by using the term "distress." The NCCN (2008) has created the Distress Thermometer, a VAS (0–10, 0 = no distress, 10 = extreme distress) and described significant distress as ≥4. The NCCN tool also includes a checklist of specific concerns causing distress; for example, practical concerns such as financial issues and family concerns including dealing with children, emotional concerns such as depression and fears, and physical concerns, such as fatigue and pain. The Distress Thermometer may provide a general measure of overall distress as well more detailed information about the specific concerns. This allows oncology nurses to accurately assess and document the survivor's experience and target specialized referrals such as social work, psychiatry, or psychology and/or pastoral care for further assessment and interventions.

❀ Assessment for Suicidal Thoughts

Assessment for depressive signs and symptoms carries an important facet; recognizing the risk of suicidal thoughts in depressed people. Although not all people with depression contemplate suicide, it is the ethical obligation of the healthcare provider, including the oncology nurse, to assess whether a person wants to harm himself or herself. Many cancer survivors live at home with numerous, potent prescriptions that may be used to harm themselves if they are having thoughts of suicide. A history of depression, previous suicide attempts, substance abuse, and/or recent loss put a person at higher risk for suicidal thoughts. A few targeted questions can be used to assess for suicidal thoughts. An answer of yes to any of these questions requires rapid referral for further assessment and interventions by specialized providers. Questions such as the following may be useful for opening up this difficult topic area with depressed people and promoting discussion and evaluation:

- Most people with cancer have passing thoughts about suicide, such as, "I might do something if it gets bad enough." Have you ever had thoughts like that?
- Any thoughts of not wanting to live, or wishing your illness might hasten your death?
- Do you have thoughts of suicide? Have you thought about how you would do it? Do you intend to harm yourself? (Adapted from NCI, 2009; Roth & Holland, 1995)

⑧ Interventions

Oncology nurses can assess for the presence of depression in cancer survivors by performing brief assessments at routine visits. These assessments provide valuable information about the survivor's mental health without directly providing counseling interventions. However, by asking these questions, the nurse often opens the door, allowing survivors to discuss their concerns. Although sometimes nurses fear that opening up these discussions will either make things worse or allow the person to talk about topics the nurse may not feel able to handle or have the time to properly address, these discussions are therapeutic in themselves, increasing trust and allowing disclosure of concerns. Deciding on the next steps after one of these discussions depends on the cancer survivor's level of depression and the nurse's comfort with the revelations. If the nurse feels comfortable providing support and referring the more depressed patient for further evaluation, then those are appropriate interventions. If the oncology nurse is unsure what the person's responses may mean about the survivor's overall experience and mental health, then consultation with a colleague and/or referral are in order. When oncology nurses express concern and acknowledge survivors' experiences, then it is more likely that they will be receptive to counseling and/or pharmacologic interventions if needed.

A statement such as the following can follow one of these discussions if the survivor appears to need further evaluation:

> *Many people with cancer sometimes have these feelings. You are not alone. But talking to someone else about them can greatly help. I'd like to suggest that you consider doing that. Would you be willing to talk to someone who has a lot of experience helping people cope with the stress of having cancer? (NCI, 2009).*

Interventions for depression depend on the nature and severity of the signs and symptoms as well as risk factors and medical conditions and other treatments. According to the Oncology Nursing Society's (ONS) Putting Evidence into Practice® (PEP) Team on Depression, there is sufficient evidence in the literature to recommend that all patients be screened for depression at every visit. People at high risk for depression should be referred to specialized services to prevent the development of significant distress, including depression. Interventions that have the highest level of evidence are psychoeducational and psychosocial interventions, including cognitive behavioral therapy, patient education, counseling and psychotherapy, behavioral therapy, and supportive interventions (Fulcher *et al.*, 2008).

The recommendations of the ONS PEP Team on Depression follow:

- Refer high-risk patients to specialized psychological services to minimize the likelihood of developing significant distress.
- Use a range of psychoeducational interventions to decrease distress.
- Manage depression by incorporating a combination of supportive psychotherapy, cognitive and behavioral techniques, and pharmacotherapy.
- There is no evidence that any particular antidepressant is superior to another in the management of depression in people with cancer.
- Other therapies that may improve depression are art, music, painting, reading, poetry, wellness programs, meditation, hypnosis, acupuncture, relaxation, exercise, prayer, laughter, etc..

Psychosocial and psychoeducational interventions are frequently within the scope of nursing practice and are integral to providing high-quality nursing care in oncology. These interventions include cognitive behavioral therapy, patient education and information, counseling and psychotherapy, behavioral therapy, and supportive interventions (Fulcher *et al.*, 2008). Although these interventions vary in their type and frequency, there is sufficient evidence in the literature that they reduce depressive symptoms in adults during and after cancer treatment.

Pharmacologic Agents

Pharmacologic agents are frequently used to treat depression and also have a role in treating cancer survivors. In the *Clinical Practice Guidelines for the Psychosocial Care of Adults with Cancer* (2003), treatment for depression in adults with cancer should include both psychotherapeutic interventions and pharmacologic agents. Although there is no evidence that one antidepressant medication works better than another, the medication should be based on the side effect profile and the patient's needs. See a specific pharmacologic text for review of the different antidepressants and/or consult a healthcare provider with specialization in prescribing pharmacologic agents.

Antidepressant medications used in people with cancer include:

- Selective serotonin reuptake inhibitors (SSRIs), such as fluoxetine (Prozac), fluvoxamine (Luvox), Sertraline (Zoloft), paroxetine (Paxil), Citalopram (Celexa), and escitalopram (Lexapro)
- Tricyclic antidepressants (TCAs), such as amitriptyline (Elavil), imipramine (Tofranil), desipramine (Norpramin), nortriptyline (Pamelor), and doxepin (Sinequan)
- Serotonin–norepinephrine reuptake inhibitors (SNRIs), such as venlafaxine (Effexor) and duloxetine (Cymbalta)
- Other antidepressants, such as mirtazapine (Remeron), bupropion (Wellbutrin), and trazodone (Desyrel)

Other Nonpharmacologic Interventions

Nonpharmacologic interventions may also be useful in relieving depressive symptoms in people with cancer. Exercise has increasingly been shown to be useful in relieving anxiety and depression in people with cancer, particularly in studies of patients with breast cancer. In the ONS PEP review of the literature, relaxation therapy with or without guided imagery, hypnosis and autogenic training has been found to decrease feelings of distress and depression (Fulcher *et al.*, 2008). Additionally, massage therapy and hypnotherapy have also been evaluated for their effectiveness in relieving depressive symptoms with insufficient evidence.

New Directions

Earlier research on depression in people with cancer focused on the negative aspects of the impact of a cancer diagnosis and explored whether this event was similar to a responses to a traumatic event such as posttraumatic stress syndrome. Newer research has moved into the role of benefit-finding; that is, looking for the positive to promote growth and well-being in people facing cancer. Stimulants such as methylphenidate (Ritalin and Concerta) have also shown some efficacy in relieving depression in people with advanced cancer. Longitudinal research is needed to follow long-term survivors and understand their experience and identify points of increased vulnerability for depression and effective interventions.

Summary

Oncology nurses are an integral part of the oncology team when caring for cancer survivors. As more people with cancer are surviving for years after treatment, it is the oncology nurse who frequently has contact with survivors and their families. Their knowledge about survivors' previous experiences and family relationships is valuable in understanding survivors' experiences during follow-up. There is little evidence regarding the long-term effects of a cancer diagnosis and treatment on mental health, including the development of depression years after initial treatment or during long-term adjuvant therapies. Oncology nurses are trained to assess, support, and refer their patients if signs of depression develop during survivorship. Their relationships with survivors are often based on trust, facilitating the disclosure of emotional concerns that require further assessment and perhaps interventions. Supportive interventions such as teaching and supportive responses are often effective in addressing concerns, normalizing the experience, and relieving symptoms of depression. Oncology nurses are also ideally suited to observe changes in concerns and levels of distress, and offer support to survivors and referral to other healthcare providers for intensive interventions.

References

American Psychiatric Association. (1994). *Diagnostic and statistical manual of mental disorders* (4th ed.). Washington, DC: Author.

Beck, A. T. (1972). *Depression: Causes and treatment*. Philadelphia: University of Pennsylvania Press.

Beck, A. T., Steer, R. A., & Garbin, M. G. (1988). Psychometric properties of Beck Depression Inventory: Twenty-five years of evaluation. *Clinical Psychology Review, 8,* 77–100.

Derogatis, L. R., Morrow, G. R., Fetting, J., Penman, D., Piasetsky, S., Schmale, A. M., *et al.* (1983). The prevalence of psychiatric disorders among cancer patients. *Journal of the American Medical Association, 249,* 751.

Fulcher, C. D., Badger, T., Gunter, A. K., Marrs, J. A., & Reese, J. M. (2008). Putting Evidence into Practice (PEP): Depression. *Clinical Journal of Oncology Nursing, 12*(1), 131–140.

National Cancer Institute. (2009). Depression PDQ: Assessment and diagnosis. Retrieved January 22, 2009, from http://www.cancer.gov/cancertopics/pdq/supportivecare/depression/HealthProfessional/356.cdr#Section_356

National Comprehensive Cancer Network. (2008). *NCCN clinical practice guidelines in oncology*™: *Distress management* [v.1.2008]. Retrieved January 21, 2009, from http://www.nccn.org/professionals/physician_gls/PDF/distress.pdf

Payne, D. K., & Massie, M. J. (2002). Anxiety and depression. In A. M. Berger, R, K, Portenoy, & D. E. Weissman (Eds.), *Principles of palliative care and supportive oncology* (2nd ed., p. 577). Philadelphia: Lippincott Williams & Wilkins.

Roth, A. J., & Holland, J. C. (1995). Psychiatric complications in cancer patients. In M. C., Brain & P. P., Carbone, (Eds.), *Current therapy in hematology-oncology* (5th ed.) St. Louis: Mosby-Year Book, 609–618.

Zabora, J., Britzenhofeszoc, K., Curbow, B., Hooker, C., & Piantadosi, S. (2001). The prevalence of psychological distress by cancer site. *Psychooncology, 10,* 19–28.

Zigmond, A. S., & Snaith, R. P. (1983). The hospital anxiety and depression scale. *Acta Psychiatria Scandanavia, 67,* 361–370.

Bibliography

Badger, T. (2008). *Evidence-based outcomes measurement summaries—Depression.* Oncology Nursing Society. Retrieved July 23, 2008, from http://www.ons.org/outcomes/measures/depression.shtml

National Health and Medical Research Council, Australia. (2003). *Clinical practice guidelines for the psychosocial care of adults with cancer.* Retrieved January 23, 2009, from http://www.nhmrc.gov.au/publications/synopses/cp90syn.htm

❀ SLEEP DISTURBANCES IN CANCER SURVIVORS

Wendy E. Bayles-Dazet

❀ Introduction

Few people can claim to have *never* had a restless night's sleep. However, there is growing appreciation for the importance of a restful night's sleep for cancer survivors and their caregivers. Sleep medicine is a burgeoning science that has practical applications for many in this population. This section provides a brief overview of the cycles of sleep, and discusses the interaction between sleep problems and some common outcomes. Lastly, evidence-based practice interventions that may help to reverse common sleeping problems are discussed in an attempt to provide the seriously ill patient, survivors, and their caregivers with some welcome relief and rest.

❀ Normal Sleep Patterns

Normal sleep consists of two distinct states: non-rapid eye movement (NREM) and rapid eye movement (REM). The bulk of a typical 8-hour sleep period consists primarily of NREM sleep. The four stages of NREM sleep are:

- Stage 1 (5–10% of total sleep)
- Stage 2 (50% of total sleep)
- Stages 3 and 4 are slow wave, or delta, sleep (20% of total sleep)

REM sleep occurs at the end of Stage 4 sleep. The cycle continues throughout the night, although REM periods are significantly longer and deeper during the second half of the night. The sleep–wake cycle is part of the body's overall circadian rhythm. Timing of this cycle is intricately involved with other biological rhythms, such as autonomic changes in pulse and blood pressure, and the release of various hormones. Ventilatory response to hypercapnia and hypoxemia is diminished during REM sleep; this can result in hypoventilation in susceptible individuals (Sateia & Byock, 2009).

Proper sleep provides a restorative function in the body. This is contingent on a number of factors, such as adequate physical comfort (i.e., cool temperatures, darkened room, lack of pain, absence of psychological distress). Unfortunately, any alterations in an individual's "sleep architecture" (cycles of sleep) can impact the quality of his or her life. With advancing age, there is a tendency toward lighter sleep. It often becomes increasingly fragmented when complicated by medical and mental health conditions.

⑧ Sleep Disturbances and Cancer

Many previous reports have pointed out the high prevalence of sleep disturbances in cancer patients (Savard & Morin, 2001; Sela, 2005). Psychological distress, particularly depression and anxiety, may contribute to insomnia and complaints of daytime fatigue (Mystakidou *et al.*, 2006). Pain regulation is often contingent on sleep quality. A study investigating the influence of cancer-related pain on various QOL indicators revealed that 58% of cancer patients awoke during the night because of pain (Strang & Qvarner, 1990). Pain intensity has also been demonstrated to correlate inversely with total hours of sleep in patients with advanced cancer (Tamburini, Selmi, DeConno, & Ventafridda, 1987). Quality of sleep also appears to be associated with immune function. A recent study showed an increase in interferon-gamma and IL-1 beta after cognitive-behavioral therapy for insomnia in cancer patients (Savard, Simard, Ivers, & Morin, 2005).

Sleepiness must be distinguished from more general and vague complaints of tiredness and fatigue, which are common among people dealing with cancer. Cognitive function can be reduced when the ability to pay attention and retain information is compromised as a result of sleep disturbance. Depression, irritability, and social withdrawal can also be potential complications of sleep disturbance. Patients who are sleepy tend to be inactive, less motivated, and less capable of participating in treatment (Sateia & Byock, 2009). Physical sequelae of inactivity can precipitate a heightened risk for deep vein thrombosis, pulmonary emboli, and decubitus ulcers.

Assessment

It is important for healthcare providers to recognize the importance of a good night's sleep in this population, and routinely ask their patients about how they are sleeping at night. It's also important to inquire about daytime sleepiness and other related sleep–wake disturbances; i.e., restless leg syndrome, snoring, and sleep apnea (an absence of respiration that can last anywhere from 10 seconds to 2–3 minutes, which is especially relevant in patients with head and neck cancers), parasomnias (e.g., sleepwalking/talking, sleep paralysis, night terrors), or narcolepsy (excessive daytime sleepiness).

The most widely used sleep-specific questionnaire is the Pittsburgh Sleep Quality Index (PSQI) (Buysse, Reynolds, Monk, Berman, & Kupfer, 1989). The questionnaire measures subjective sleep quality during the previous month. Scoring is accomplished by adding up the scores on sleep quality, sleep latency, sleep duration, habitual sleep efficiency, sleep disturbances, sleeping medication usage, and daytime dysfunction. A score of greater than 8 points indicates that the patient is a poor sleeper. Other objective instruments can include sleep diaries that can be provided for the patient to complete, and then hand back in after a week's time. Sometimes a day log can be provided as well, to record events and emotions that might contribute to poor sleep patterns. With more severe cases, an overnight stay in a sleep lab utilizes polysomnography to determine the quality of the sleep architecture.

In a longitudinal study comparing symptom experiences in men and women with inoperable lung cancer, Lovgren, Tishelman, Sprangers, (2008) compared the prevalence and intensity of different symptoms at three time points: close to diagnosis, at 1 month, and at 3 months. At all three time points, fatigue was listed as the most prominent symptom. For men, the most common symptom at all time reports was sleep disturbance; for women, sleep disturbance was reported more commonly at the first two time points. Prevalence and intensity of sleep disturbance improved over time. Emotional function was scored at its worst when closest to diagnosis; this was likely influenced by sleep quality as well.

Another study focused on sleep patterns in patients with advanced lung cancer prior to chemotherapy. The sleep quality of advanced lung cancer patients versus matched controls with obstructive sleep apnea was examined. The lung cancer patients had significantly poorer sleep, more daytime sleepiness, and lower QOL scores. Almost all lung cancer patients (96%) were reported to have sleep dysfunction scores greater than that seen in the normal population. They were also twice as likely to use sleep medications in the past months (31.6% vs 15.4%). These scores may be a result of comorbid conditions such as emphysema; however, no data were available about tobacco use, so results were inconclusive (Gooneratne *et al.*, 2007).

⊗ Treatment

Treatments for sleep disorders have historically included sedative-hypnotics, such as chloral hydrate and barbiturates; however, these came with increased risk of dependence as well as a risk of death with overdose. In the 1960s, tricyclic antidepressants (i.e., amitriptyline, doxepin) showed the side effect of sedation, and so were used for insomnia. However, these medications had cardiac side effects, anticholinergic effects, and daytime sedation. The benzodiazepines (i.e., triazolam, flurazepam, temazepam), came into favor in the mid-1960s and were preferred for their overdose safety. Unfortunately, they also had abuse potential, could cause daytime sedation, and reportedly were associated with memory impairment.

In 1980, trazodone (a heterocyclic antidepressant) began to be used more often to treat insomnia than for depression. It was perceived as having less abuse and dependence potential than the benzodiazepines. There are very little data supporting the efficacy of trazodone. Side effects can include daytime sedation/hangover, orthostatic hypotension, and the risk of priapism. In the late 1990s, the nonbenzodiazepines were introduced (i.e., zolpidem, zaleplon, eszopiclone). These medications have shown to be "efficacious in the short-term management of insomnia" (National Institutes of Health, 2005). However, this report also notes that adverse effects can include residual sedation, cognitive impairment, dependence, motor incoordination, and rebound insomnia. Some over-the-counter and herbal preparations have been used to treat insomnia, such as valerian extract, melatonin, and diphenhydramine; however, large-scale studies have not been conducted and some degree of caution still seems advisable.

Recent years have shown an increase in behavioral models for treating chronic insomnia. The cognitive–behavioral approach works to correct or remove perpetuating mechanisms that maintain or contribute to poor sleep patterns. Sleep hygiene suggests:

- Scrupulous attention to bed times and awakening times
- Limiting caffeine, nicotine, and alcohol
- No exercise after 6 PM

- Limiting bed use for sleep and sexual activity
- Optimizing the sleep environment: low light, noise, temperature

Relaxation therapies have also been introduced as a means to reduce arousal, including progressive muscle relaxation, guided imagery, meditation, and/or biofeedback. These techniques are often more suited for sleep-onset difficulties versus mid-cycle awakenings.

Good clinical practice would suggest that a careful assessment of the cancer patient's subjective assessment of his or her sleep quality, somatic and psychological complaints, type of cancer, and concomitant medications would prove valuable in determining which treatment modality to use. A sophisticated behavioral model known as Sleep Restriction Therapy was developed by Spielman, Saskin, and Thorpy (1987), which incorporated a logarithm of sleep efficiency by either increasing or decreasing time in bed in an attempt to restore homeostatic drive.

As knowledge of sleep disorders and their treatments grows, it becomes increasingly clear that there is a connection between quality of sleep and corresponding psychological coping, and immunologic and cognitive functioning. Current literature underscores the relationship between insomnia and correlates such as depression, pain, and fatigue. It is important to include the caregiver in the dialogue about quality of sleep. Sleep disruption as a result of grief, anxiety, and depression were frequently cited among relatives of cancer patients (Sawyer, Antoniou, Toogood, Rice, & Baghurst, 1994). Additionally, care providers may have frequent nighttime disruptions that contribute to psychophysiologic insomnia, a condition marked by the inability to reach restorative sleep because of hypervigilance. This, in turn, can result in fatigue and subsequent depression. Both cancer survivors and their partners and caregivers should be assessed for sleep disturbances that may affect the well-being and functioning of both.

❀ Summary

In conclusion, the last several decades have shown a growing recognition on the part of clinicians that attention to survivors' and caregivers' sleep is an essential aspect of good clinical care in the cancer population. Problems relating to sleep have been shown to be the most prevalent concern in people who are seriously ill. Achieving a good night's sleep can have implications for one's ability to cope, as well as in promoting efficient immunologic functioning. It can provide much-needed respite from worries and physical discomforts, and restore hope to both the cancer survivor and caregiver. Therefore, it is vitally important that oncology nurses and other healthcare providers address sleep quality during all phases of treatment. Recognition and treatment of sleep disruptions is likely to improve outcomes for survivors and their caregivers, and may even reduce complicated grieving patterns in future.

References

Buysse, D. J., Reynolds, C. F. 3rd, Monk, T. H., Berman, S. R., & Kupfer, D. J. (1989). The Pittsburgh Sleep Quality Index: A new instrument for psychiatric practice and research. *Psychiatry Research, 28,* 193–213.

Gooneratne, N. S., Dean, G. E., Rogers, A. E., Nkwuo, J. E., Coyne, J. C., & Kaiser, L. R. (2007). Sleep and quality of life in long-term lung cancer survivors. *Lung Cancer, 58,* 403–410.

Lovgren, M., Tishelman, C., Sprangers, M., Kovi, H., & Hamberg, K. (2008). Symptoms and problems with functioning among women and men with inoperable lung cancer: a longitudinal study. *Lung Cancer, 60,* 113–124.

Mystakidou, K., Tsilika, E., Parpa, E., Katsouda, E., Galanos, A., & Vlahos, L. (2006). Psychological distress of patients with advanced cancer: Influence and contribution of pain severity and pain interference. *Cancer Nursing, 10*(2), 85–92.

National Institutes of Health. (2005). State of the Science Report: Chronic Insomnia. Retrieved February 17, 2009, from http://consensus.nih.gov/2005/2005InsomniaSOS026html.htm

Sateia, M. & Byock, I. (2009). Sleep in palliative care. In: *Oxford Textbook of Palliative Medicine,* 4th Edition. G. Hanks, N. Cherny, N. Christakas, M. Fallon, S. Kaasa, R. Portenoy. (Eds.) Oxford University Press, Oxford. In press.

Savard, J., & Morin, C. M. (2001). Insomnia in the context of cancer: A review of a neglected problem. *Journal of Clinical Oncology, 19,* 895–908.

Savard, J., Simard, S., Ivers, H., & Morin, C. M. (2005). Randomized study on the efficacy of cognitive-behavioral therapy for insomnia secondary to breast cancer, part I: Sleep and psychological effects. *Journal of Clinical Oncology, 23*(25), 6083–6096.

Sawyer, M. G., Antoniou, G., Toogood, I., Rice, M., & Baghurst, P. A. (1994). A prospective study of the psychological adjustment of parents and families of children with cancer. *Journal of Paediatric and Child Health, 29*(5), 352–356.

Sela, R. A., Watanabe, S., & Nekolaichuk, C. L. (2005). Sleep disturbances in palliative cancer patients attending a pain and symptom control clinic. *Palliative and Supportive Care, 3,* 23–31.

Spielman, A. J., Saskin, P., & Thorpy, M. J. (1987). Treatment of chronic insomnia by restriction of time in bed. *Sleep,* 10, 45–55.

Strang, P., & Qvarner, H. (1990). Cancer-related pain and its influence on quality of life. *Anticancer Research, 10,* 1, 109–112.

Tamburini, M., Selmi, S., DeConno, F., & Ventafridda, V. (1987). Semantic descriptors of pain. *Pain, 29*(2), 187–193.

Bibliography

Carter, P. A., & Chang, B. L. (2000). Sleep and depression in cancer caregivers. *Cancer Nursing, 23,* 6, 410–5.

Hauri, P., & Linde, S. (1996). *No more sleepless nights.* New York: John Wiley & Sons.

Irwin, M. R., Wang, M., Campomayor, C. O., Collado-Hidalgo, A., & Cole, S. (2006). Sleep deprivation and activation of morning levels of cellular and genomic markers of inflammation. *Archives in Internal Medicine, 166,* 16, 1756–1762.

Sateia, M., & Lang, B. (2008). Sleep and cancer: Recent developments. *Current Oncology Reports 10*(4), 309–318.

Savard, J., Miller, S. M., Mills, M., *et al.* (1999). Association between subjective sleep quality and depression on immunocompetence in low-income women at risk for cervical cancer. *Psychosomatic Medicine, 61,* 4, 496–507.

CULTURE AND CANCER SURVIVORSHIP

Wendye DiSalvo and Laura Urquhart

Introduction

Culture is a vital and fundamental aspect of being human, and culture care must be addressed and acknowledged. As healthcare professionals, knowledge and understanding about cultures is paramount in order to assist individuals of different cultures in a meaningful and beneficial way. Culture may be defined as "the learned and shared beliefs, values and life ways of a designated or particular group which are generally transmitted intergenerationally and influences one's thinking and action modes" (Leininger, 1995, p. 9). Culture shapes how an individual develops in life. A person's culture and its unique influences can predict reaction to life stressors, especially illness. When a life-changing event, such as the diagnosis of cancer, occurs, culturally competent care should include recognition of multiple factors, such as ethnicity, gender, sexual orientation, and social class. These factors have significant influence on communication with healthcare providers, family, and friends. Clearly, the identification of culture and its value for the survivor can influence health. Healthcare providers who show a degree of culture awareness convey respect for cultural diversity.

There are more cancer survivors whose survival and living with the sequelae of treatment is colored by their individual culture. For example, until recently in Japan, Japanese patients would not be told their diagnosis by the physician, as they believed this information would harm the patient's QOL (Yamaguchi, 2002). The consequential meaning of survivorship may vary according to the culture and be defined by what QOL means in that culture (Findley, 2007).

The perception of QOL, spirituality, and family varies by culture and ethnicity. Chaturvedi (1991) found that QOL, as it related to spirituality, was more important than individual functioning in Indian cancer patients, families, and caregivers. In cancer patients who were of Mexican descent, QOL was equated with happiness, being active and connected to their families. Families of Mexican descent often try to hide a diagnosis of cancer, believing the person will die sooner if he or she knows (Feurerstein, 2007; Juarez, Ferrell & Borneman, 1998). Studies conducted in the Chinese culture found that gynecologic cancer survivors felt the cause of their disease was related to an imbalance in the Yin and Yang related to sexual activity. Beliefs about cancer were influenced by education, patriarchal family structure, and the subservient role of women in the culture. Important survivorship QOL issues were mobility, accepting one's position, social support, and being able to eat (Findley, 2007; Molassiotis, Chan, Yam, Chan, & Lam, 2002). Beliefs and perceptions in the Chinese culture concerning cancer include cancer is infectious; related to excessive activities; gynecologic cancers may reoccur if they engage in further sexual activity; and traditional healers are an important part of restoring balance in the patient's life (Chan *et al.*, 2002; Findley, 2007).

In looking at statistical data, it is clear that disparities exist among different ethnic groups and regionally in the United States. Ethnic and racial minority populations tend to present for treatment at later stages of cancer and have higher mortality rates from cancer (American Cancer Society, 2006). Factors known to contribute to racial disparities vary by cancer site and include difference in exposure to underlying risk factors (e.g., historical smoking prevalence for lung cancer among men), access to high-quality regular screening (breast, cervical, and colorectal cancer), and timely diagnosis and treatment. These data support the need for vital state and federal programs that offer free screening. The higher breast cancer incidence rates among whites are thought to reflect a combination of factors that affect both diagnosis (e.g., mammography in white women), and the underlying factors that affect disease occurrence (e.g., later age of first birth, and greater use of hormonal replacement therapy among white compared with African-American women) (Jemal *et al.*, 2008). Racial and ethnic minorities tend to receive lower-quality health care than whites, even when insurance status, income, age and severity of conditions are comparable (ACS, 2006).

In the United States, disparities in cancer are well documented. In order to reduce health disparities, there needs to be an effective use of social and cultural constructs to communicate about health and behaviors that can reduce risks of developing cancer and lead to earlier diagnosis.

⊗ Summary

Culture is a commanding influence on the way individuals envision the world, and make choices and decisions that guide their actions. Awareness of disparities is essential in advocating for screening, early treatment and follow-up. Oncology nurses' awareness of cultural influences and preferences, values, and practices can facilitate care and improve patient and family outcomes.

References

American Cancer Society. (2006). *Cancer facts and figures for African Americans: 2005–2006.* Atlanta: The American Cancer Society.

Chan, Y. M., Ngan, H. Y., Yip, P. S., Li, B. Y., Lau, O. W., & Tang, G. W. (2001). Psychological adjustment in gynecological cancers survivors: A longitudinal study on risk factors for maladjustment. *Gynecological Oncology*, *80*(3), 387–3394.

Chaturvedi, S. K. (1991). What's important for quality of life to Indians in relation to cancer. *Social Science Medicine*, *33*(1), 91–94.

Feuerstein, M., Ed. (2007). *Handbook of cancer survivorship.* New York: Springer.

Findley, P. A. (2007). Global considerations. In M. Feuerstein, (Ed.) *Handbook of cancer survivorship* (pp. 449–479). New York: Springer.

Jemal, A., Siegel, R., Ward, E., Hao, Y., Xu, J., Murray, T., *et al.* (1998). Cancer statistic. *CA: A Journal for Clinicians*, *58*(?), 71–96.

Juarez, G., Ferrell, B., & Borneman, T. (1998). Perceptions of quality of life in Hispanic patients with cancer. *Cancer Practice*, *6*(6), 318–324.

Leininger, M. (1995). *Transcultural nursing concepts: Theories, research & practices* (2nd ed.). New York: McGraw-Hill.

Molassiotis, A., Chan, C. W., Yam, B. M., Chan, S. J., & Lam, C. S. (2002). Life after cancer: Adaptation issues faced by Chinese gynecological cancer survivors in Hong Kong. *Psycho-Oncology, 11*(2), 114–123.

Yamaguchi, K. (2002). Overview of cancer control programs in Japan. *Japanese Journal of Oncology, 32*(31), 22–31.

Bibliography

Curtiss, C. P., & Haylock. P. J. (2006). Managing late and long-term sequelae of cancer and cancer treatment. *American Journal of Nursing, 106,* (Suppl 3), 22–23.

🕮 DYSPNEA

Wendye DiSalvo

🕮 Introduction

Dyspnea is a distressing symptom for many cancer survivors. It has been defined as "a subjective experience of breathing discomfort that consists of qualitatively distinct sensations that vary in intensity." The experience of dyspnea has been difficult to quantify because it arises from "multiple physiological, psychological, social and environmental factors, and may induce secondary physiological and behavioral responses" (American Thoracic Society, 1999). Dyspnea may directly affect QOL and is not always amenable to healthcare interventions (Disalvo, Joyce, Tyson, Culkin, & Mackay, 2008).

A significant number of cancer patients are affected by this symptom. As many as 15–55% of patients are affected by dyspnea at diagnosis. It is also a common and distressing symptom at the end of life, occurring in 18–79% of patients (Ripamonti & Fusco, 2002). Because oncology nurses frequently are involved in the care of patients during treatment and follow-up, they can also assess for dyspnea and its affects on the cancer survivor.

🕮 Assessment

Dyspnea in survivors may result from the disease, treatment or be unrelated to cancer (Dudgeon, Kristjanson, Sloan, Lentzman, & Clement, 2001). The symptom is a complex phenomenon and can be difficult to assess for multiple reasons. Dyspnea has been described as having two components: quantitative and qualitative. The quantitative element is concerned with the physiological mechanisms involved in producing the symptom. For many patients dyspnea is the result of stimulation of a variety of mechanoreceptors in the upper airway, lungs, and chest wall and is responsible for sensations that arise when there is a mechanical load on the system. Derangement in oxygenation and/or acidemia can lead to breathing discomfort and has the potential for amelioration (Scano & Ambrosino, 2002). Common causes of dyspnea that are unrelated to cancer include chronic obstructive pulmonary disease (COPD), asthma, interstitial lung disease and myocardial dysfunction pneumothorax, obesity, and aspiration (Scano & Ambrosino, 2002). Dyspnea can be an indirect result of cancer from conditions including anemia, pneumonia, electrolyte imbalance, cachexia, pulmonary emboli, and ascites. Treatment-related dyspnea may be caused by surgery, radiation, and chemotherapy-induced pulmonary toxicity cardiomyopathy. Cancer-related dyspnea may arise from primary or metastatic cancer to the lung, pleural tumor, lymphangitic carcinomatosis, pericardial effusion, superior vena cava syndrome, paraneoplastic syndrome, hepatomegaly, pulmonary leukostasis, and/or tumor burden (McDermott, 2000). Whatever the underlying cause, the quality of life in cancer patients can be adversely impacted by the symptom of dyspnea (Smith *et al.*, 2001).

The qualitative component of dyspnea relies on the survivor's perspective of breathlessness. A visual analog scale (VAS) can be used to assess the degree of breathlessness experienced by cancer survivors. Repeated use of the VAS provides information as to the symptom's intensity and changes in dyspnea over time (Hately, Laurence, Scott, Baker, & Thomas, 2003).

Treatment

Oncology nurses are in a unique position to advocate for the treatment of this distressing symptom for survivors and families. If the underlying cause of dyspnea is identified, then appropriate measures can be initiated to minimize the distress. The ONS has provided oncology nurses with PEP® cards regarding common symptoms found in cancer patients and the nursing interventions that may be effective in relieving the symptoms. A PEP card was developed for dyspnea, providing evidence-based interventions that are within the scope of nursing practice or are essential to nursing care in collaboration with the healthcare team.

The following are interventions listed on the PEP card:

- Opioids, in both oral and parental forms, were found to be effective in relieving the breathless sensation in patients with terminal or advanced cancer. Short-acting or parental opioids decrease ventilatory demand by decreasing central respiratory drive. The most frequently used short-acting opioid in the literature was morphine. The dose is dependent on whether the patient is opioid naïve or already using narcotics for other reasons (Disalvo *et al.*, 2008; Jennings, Davis, Higgins, Gibbs, & Broadley, 2002). The effectiveness of using nebulized opioids is not established (Joyce, McSweeney, Carrieri-Kohlman, & Hawkins, 2004).
- Supplemental oxygen use in hypoxic patients with dyspnea at rest was valuable in relieving the symptom (Bruera *et al.*, 1993).
- Nonpharmacological interventions that have been employed but not yet proven to be effective include acupuncture and cognitive behavioral approach.
- Cognitive behavioral interventions and breathing retraining have been useful in combination with nurse-delivered psychosocial support interventions (Hately *et al.*, 2003).
- Both the acupuncture and cognitive behavioral approach reported improvement in symptoms but need further research with well-designed studies.

The National Comprehensive Cancer Network (NCCN, 2006) published Clinical Practice Guidelines that were developed by a committee of experts utilizing clinical expertise and accessible scientific evidence. These guidelines are based on the individual life expectancy and address treating the underlying cause of the symptom and/or comorbid condition. An example would be a thoracentesis for a significant pleural effusion in an individual who had years to months to live. In the patient with months to weeks to live, the guidelines include the use of benzodiazepines for anxiety and the use of opioids for dyspnea and/or cough as well as nonpharmacological measures. The use of support, stress reduction, relaxation techniques, fans, and cooler temperatures are recommended. For the dying patient the following is indicated: management of secretions with medications, use of oxygen therapy, withholding or withdrawing mechanical ventilation as indicated by patient and family, sedation, management of fluid overload, and anticipatory guidance and support for dying patients and their families.

❧ Summary

There is an important opportunity for nursing research for this distressing and debilitating symptom in cancer patients. Short-acting opioids are beneficial in ameliorating the symptom of dyspnea. Alternative, complementary, and nonpharmacological interventions showed promise but the studies have been small sample sizes. Implementation of evidence-based interventions by oncology nurses will improve outcomes for survivors and their families.

References

American Thoracic Society. (1999). Dyspnea. Mechanisms, assessment, and management: A consensus statement. *American Journal of Respiratory and Critical Care Medicine, 159,* 321–340.

Bruera, E., de Stoutz, N., Velasco-Leiva, A., Schoeller, T., & Hanson, J. (1993). Effects of oxygen on dyspnea in hypoxaemic terminal-cancer patients. *Lancet, 342*(8862), 13–14.

DiSalvo, W. M., Joyce, M. M., Tyson, L.B., Culkin, A. E., & Mackay, K. M. (2008). Putting evidence into practice: Evidence based interventions for cancer-related dyspnea. *Clinical Journal of Oncology Nursing, 12*(2), 341–352.

Dudgeon, D. J., Kristjanson, L., Sloan, J.A., Lertzman, M., & Clement, K. (2001). Dyspnea in cancer patients: Prevalence and Associated factors, *Journal of Pain and Symptom Management, 21*(2), 95–102.

Hately, J., Laurence, V., Scott, A., Baker, R., & Thomas, P. (2003). Breathlessness clinics within specialist palliative care settings can improve the quality of life and functional capacity of patients with lung cancer. *Palliative Medicine, 17*(5), 410–417.

Jennings, A. L., Davies, A. N., Higgins, J. P. T., Gibbs, J. S. R., & Broadley K. E. (2002). A systematic review of the use of opioids in the management of dyspnoea. *Thorax, 57,* 939–944.

Joyce, M., McSweeney, M., Carrieri- Kohlman, K. I., & Hawkins, J. (2004). The use of nebulized opioids in the management of dyspnea: Evidence synthesis. *Oncology Nursing Forum, 3*(13), 551–561.

McDermott, M. K. (2000) Dyspnea. In D. Camp-Sorrell & R. A. Hawkins (Eds.). *Clinical manual for the oncology advance practice nurse* (pp. 131–135). Pittsburgh, PA: Oncology Nursing Press, Inc.

Ripamonti, C., & Fusco, F. (2002). Respiratory problems in advanced cancer. *Supportive Care in Cancer, 10*(3), 204–216.

Scano, G., & Ambrosino, N. (2002). Pathophysiology of dyspnea. *Lung, 180*(3), 131–148.

Smith, E. L., Hann, D. M, Ahles, T. A., Furstenberg, C. T., Mitchell, T. A., Meyer, L., *et al.* (2001). Dyspnea, anxiety and body consciousness, and quality of life in patients with lung cancer. *Journal of Pain and Symptom Management, 21*(4), 323–329.

Bibliography

National Comprehensive Cancer Network. (2006). Clinical practice guidelines in oncology: Palliative care. Retrieved on February 3, 2009, from http://www.nccn.org/professionals/physician_gls/PDF/palliative.pdf

❀ COGNITIVE DYSFUNCTION

Laura Urquhart

One of the most complex and challenging late side effects of cancer treatment is neurocognitive deficits. Interest in the neuropsychological impact of cancer treatment dates back to 1983, when Silberfarb and colleagues observed a measurable cognitive decline among patients undergoing cancer treatment. In the 1990s, greater recognition of chemotherapy-related cognitive dysfunction occurred (Van Dam *et al.*, 1998, Wieneke & Dienst, 1995).

Chemo brain is the term many survivors use to describe their dysfunction in memory and attention. Some remark that they just do not think the same as they did prior to chemotherapy treatment in relation to memory and organization.

Clinicians experience difficulty in assessing true cognitive dysfunction versus contributing factors or confounding cognitive dysfunction. Because cognitive dysfunction may be caused by many factors, cancer survivors should be assessed for depression, anxiety, fatigue, sleep disturbance, and hormonal effect related to cancer and its treatment. Current studies indicate that cognitive deficits, while often subtle, are observed consistently in a proportion of patients and may be durable and can be disabling (Silberfarb, 1983). Several studies have examined the effects of chemotherapy on cognition. In a study published in 1995, Wieneke and Dienst evaluated the effects of chemotherapy on breast cancer patients. Measures of working memory and sustained attention were most commonly affected.

In one study investigators compared the neuropsychologic performance of long-term survivors of breast cancer and lymphoma treated with standard-dose chemotherapy and who carried the epsilon 4 allele of the apolipoprotein E (APOE) gene to those who carry other APOE alleles. Survivors with at least one epsilon 4 allele scored significantly lower in the visual memory ($p > 0.03$) and spatial ability ($p < 0.05$), and tended to score lower in the psychomotor functioning ($p < 0.08$) as compared with survivors who did not carry an epsilon 4 allele of APOE. This gene may be a potential genetic marker for increased vulnerability to chemotherapy-induced cognitive decline (Ahles *et al.*, 2002). Clearly, there is a subset of patients who may be more vulnerable to the insult of chemotherapy on cognitive functioning.

Management

Current management of survivors who exhibit cognitive dysfunction should begin with neuropsychological assessment and include specific interventions aimed at contributing factors. After all contributing factors have been addressed, consideration should be given to cognitive rehabilitation.

Summary

Cognitive dysfunction is not fully understood. Cancer survivors represent a growing population who are at risk for the long-term consequences of their cancer diagnosis and treatment. Feuerstein (2007) notes that pharmacologic interventions and chemoprotective agents may hold promise in preventing this widespread problem, given the increasing numbers of individuals undergoing chemotherapy annually. Ferguson advocates for more research on genetic and hormonal influences and their interaction with fatigue, anxiety, and depression to discern their collective influence on function. Ultimately, the QOL for cancer survivors can be improved by assessing for cognitive dysfunction and discovering the underlying causative agents.

References

Ahles, T. A., Saykin, A. J., Furstenberg, C. T., Cole, B., Mott, L.A., & Skalla, K., et al. (2002). Neuropsychologic impact of standard dose systemic chemotherapy in long term survivors of breast cancer and lymphoma. *Journal of Clinical Oncology, 20,* 485–493.

Feuerstein, M. (2007). *Handbook of cancer survivorship.* New York: Springer Science+Business Media.

Silberfarb, P. M. (1983). Chemotherapy and cognitive deficits in cancer patients. *Annual Review in Medicine, 34,* 35–46.

Van Dam, F. S., Schagen, S. B., Muller, M. J., Boogerd, W., Wall, E., Droogleever Fortuyn, M. E., et al.(1998). Impairment of cognitive function in women receiving adjuvant treatment for high-risk breast cancer: High-dose versus standard-dose chemotherapy. *Journal of the National Cancer Institute, 90,* 210–218.

Wieneke, M. H., & Dienst, E.R. (1995). Neuropsychological assessment of cognitive functioning following chemotherapy for breast cancer. *Psycho-Oncology, 4,* 61–6.

Bibliography

Ahles, T. A., Saykin, A. J., Noll, W. W., Furstenberg, C. T., Guerin, S., Cole, B., et al. (2003). The relationship of APOE genotype to neuropsychological performance in long-term survivors treated with standard dose chemotherapy. *Psycho-Oncology, 12,* 612–619.

Barton, D., & Loprinzi, C. (2002). Novel approaches to preventing chemotherapy–induced cognitive dysfunction in breast cancer: The art of the possible. *Clinical Breast Cancer* (Suppl 3), S121–S127.

Bender, C. M., Parska, K. I., Seirika, S. M., Ryan, C. M., & Berga, S. L. (2001). Cognitive dysfunction and reproductive hormones in adjuvant therapy for breast cancer. A critical review. *Journal of Pain and Symptom Management, 21,* 407–424.

Castllon, S. A., Ganz, P. A., Bower, J. E., Peterson, L., Abraham, L., & Greendale, G. A. (2004). Neurocognitive performance in breast cancer survivors exposed to adjuvant chemotherapy and tamoxifen. *Journal of Clinical and Experiemental Neurophyschology, 26,* 955–969.

Rugo, H. S., & Ahles, T. A. (2003). The impact of adjuvant therapy for breast cancer on cognitive function: Current evidence and directions for research. *Seminars in Oncology, 30,* 749–762.

Saykin, A. J., Ahles, T. A., & McDonald, B. C. (2003). Mechanisms of chemotherapy induced cognitive dysfunction disorder: Neuropsychological pathophysiological, and neuroimaging perspectives. *Seminars in Clinical Neuropsychiatry, 8,* 201–216.

Schagen, S. B., Muller, M. J., Boogerd, W., Rosenbrand, R. M., van Rhijn, D., Rodenhuis, S., *et al.* (2002). Late effects of adjuvant chemotherapy on cognitive dysfunction: A follow up study in breast cancer patients. *Annals of Oncology, 13,* 1387–1397.

Schilling, V., Jenkins, V., Morris, R., Deutsch, D., & Bloomfield, D. (2005). The effects of adjuvant chemotherapy on cognition in women with breast cancer—preliminary results from and observational longitudinal study. *Breast, 14,* 142–150.

Tannock, I. F., Ahles, T. A., Ganz, P. A., & van Dam, F. S. (2004). Cognitive impairment associated with chemotherapy for cancer: Report of a workshop. *Journal of Clinical Oncology, 22,* 2233–2239.

Wefel, J. S., Lenzi, R., Theriault, R., Buxsar, A. U., Cruickshank, S., & Meyer, C. A. (2004). "Chemobrain" in breast carcinoma. *Cancer, 101,* 466–475.

Wefel, J. S., Lenzi, R., Theriault, R. L., Davis, R. N., & Meyers, C. A. (2004). The cognitive sequelae of standard-dose adjuvant chemotherapy in women with breast carcinoma. *Cancer, 100,* 2292–2299.

Yaffe, K., Krueger, K., Sarkar, S., Grady, D., Barret-Connor, E., Cox, D. A., *et al.* (2001). Cognitive function in postmenopausal women treated with Raloxifene. *New England Journal of Medicine, 344,* 1207–1213.

MALE SEXUALITY

Jennifer Welch and Stephanie Marcotte

Introduction

Sexuality is a normal human need throughout a person's lifetime. It is more than physical; it is also emotional, and can define our gender and sexual preferences (American Cancer Society [ACS], 1997; National Cancer Institute, 2009). With a cancer diagnosis comes physical and emotional changes that may affect sexual functioning. Survivors may experience physical or emotional issues from the disease itself or because of side effects of treatment. Common issues for men include erectile dysfunction, impaired ejaculation, loss of desire, hormone changes, body image issues, depression, and effects on fertility. These issues affect not only patients, but partners as well. This section reviews the changes related to a cancer diagnosis and treatment and their impact on male sexual functioning.

Male Sexual Function

Normal sexual function is a complex system that includes the genitalia, internal organs and neural pathways, hormone production, brain chemicals, and emotions. The testicles create sperm that is transported via the vas deferens to the seminal vesicles. The prostate gland creates semen that mixes with sperm and is transported out of the body through the urethra. This system also includes the testes that make and secrete testosterone, the adrenal gland, the pituitary gland, and hypothalamus. An erection is obtained through arousal. Orgasm creates the muscular contractions that allow for ejaculation of the semen from the vesicles down through the urethra and out of the penis (Wein, Kavoussi, Novick, Partin, & Peters, 2009).

How Cancer Diagnosis and Treatment Affects Sexuality and Sexual Dysfunction

A change in health, such as with the diagnosis of cancer, can be one of the most stressful things a person faces in a lifetime. A whole host of emotions can overwhelm a patient during this time. Often in the first stages of illness a patient is focused on understanding the disease, while undergoing rigorous diagnostic testing or surgery and making decisions about treatment options. Sexual needs sometimes rank low on the hierarchy of needs at this time. For others it provides a sense of comfort and normalcy. Each person approaches such a time and their sexuality in a unique way. Partners are also greatly affected, as they must cope with the newness and uncertainty of a cancer diagnosis while providing support to the patient (Gailbrath, Pedro, Jaffe, & Allen, 2008).

A person must continue to contend with and adjust to many changes over the course of diagnosis, treatment, and survivorship. Each phase brings new emotions and needs that may have to be met both physically and emotionally. Dysfunction can result for a variety of reasons across the survivorship spectrum (Gailbraith *et al.*, 2008).

A decreased libido, also referred to as loss of desire or sex drive, is common and may occur for many reasons. It can be caused by physical or emotional changes or a combination of both. Emotional causes are sometimes the result of the uncertainty and fear that may come with diagnosis and treatment, facing one's mortality, and the changes in roles that may occur from caregiver or provider to the one receiving care. Depression and anxiety have both emotional and physical manifestations. Physical causes are often the result of or reaction to all forms of treatment. Treatment can directly affect desire by disrupting physical function or production of hormones, but can also interfere by causing associated symptoms such as pain, nausea, vomiting, and fatigue. Body image issues can affect self-esteem and thereby impact libido.

Erectile dysfunction is a common side effect of cancer treatment. It is the inability to have and/or maintain an erection. Treatment such as surgery and radiation can cause damage to the nerves and vasculature within the penis and pelvis. Hormone disruption can occur from radiation and also androgen deprivation. Anxiety or depression can also play a role in impacting erection by altering brain chemicals, response to stimulation, and impacting emotions, and self-esteem (Wein *et al.*, 2009).

Impaired ejaculation is the inability to have an ejaculation, premature ejaculation, or dry ejaculation. Surgery can impair the nerves to the penis and pelvis interfering with one's ability to have an erection and thereby ejaculate. Dry ejaculation occurs when the prostate or other organs such as seminal vesicles or vas deferens are removed. Anxiety associated with performance can cause premature ejaculation.

Pain, sometimes referred to as dyspareunia, can result from direct treatment to genitalia, internal organs, skin, or areas of metastasis (ACS, 1997). This is not conducive to stimulation or enjoyment of sexual activity. Irritation or pain with intercourse can be noted in the urethra, prostate, scrotum, rectum, or bony structures. Every individual experiences and tolerates pain differently.

Infertility can result from surgery, radiation, chemotherapy, and hormone treatment. Surgery and radiation to the prostate, testicles, or other pelvic structures can cause direct damage to the function of organs involved in reproduction. Certain kinds of chemotherapy and whole-body radiation can cause permanent sterility. Temporary infertility may occur with hormones and external radiation.

Many surgical interventions are undertaken as part of cancer treatment. Surgery with the most impact on sexual function seems to occur in the pelvis. Nerve and vessel damage are seen with radical prostatectomy and cystectomy (Wein *et al.*, 2009). Orchiectomy impairs hormone production. Colorectal surgery, including colostomy, can cause damage to the autonomic nerves in the pelvis depending on location of tumor. Urostomy and colostomy can impact movement, comfort, and body image as well.

Patients undergoing radiation to the penis, prostate, and pelvis are at higher risk for erectile dysfunction (ED). The wider the treatment field the more risk of side effects. Dysfunction occurs because of nerve and vessel damage, scar tissue, and loss of blood vessel elasticity. Symptoms can occur acutely, but there appears to be more risk over time. One estimate states 75% of patients undergoing radiation therapy report ED 5 years after completion treatment. Testosterone disruption occurring with treatment can recover within 6 months after completion. Testosterone replacement is not usually given because of risk of contributing to recurrent prostate cancer (Wein *et al.*, 2009).

Chemotherapy may cause infertility acutely while a patient is actively on treatment. Cellular damage to sperm may be temporary, and, once chemotherapy is cleared and treatment over, a patient could pursue fertility. In high-dose chemotherapy, permanent damage is often done to sperm. Patients are encouraged to use contraception while undergoing treatment. Chemotherapy can contribute to lack of desire because of fatigue and nausea and vomiting.

Hormone therapy can decrease libido and contribute to erectile dysfunction and infertility by significantly suppressing or eliminating androgens. These hormones trigger sexual desire in the brain and play a role in fertility with production of sperm (Wein *et al.*, 2009).

Assessment of Sexual Function, Interventions, and Coping

It is important for providers to assess sexual function regularly and keep an open line of communication with patients and their partners.

A review of a patient's baseline sexual function and patient and partner expectations is helpful in assessment and treatment. A patient and partner need continued assessment, education, and information from diagnosis, through treatment, and into survivorship.

Treatment of sexual dysfunction in cancer often includes multidisciplinary team members such as primary care physician, urologist, and medical and radiation oncologist. Medications such as sildenafil citrate (Viagra), tadalafil (Cialis), and vardenafil (Levitra) may be prescribed to help with ED. Antidepressants can help to slow orgasm in premature ejaculation. Pain medication can be prescribed to help keep a patient comfortable. Surgery can be performed to repair vessel and nerve damage from treatment. Hormones can be given in situations in which treatment has affected normal production. It is rarely given to a patient with hormone-related disease such as prostate cancer. Implants can be used to preserve appearance or help with function. Penile implants help to create or maintain an erection. Testicular implants are placed to preserve the appearance of the scrotum when orchiectomy is necessary. Emotional changes can be addressed and treated in various ways. Patients and partners can be helped with both psychological and sexual counseling. Infertility can occur acutely or permanently. Sperm banking can help preserve fertility prior to treatment. Referral to fertility specialists may provide answers and options for patients. Pain specialists can treat and help manage many kinds of pain syndromes.

Despite an increase in prostate and other male cancer survivors, there is a continued lack of research on sexuality and its effect on survivorship and quality of life (Gailbraith *et al.*, 2008). There continues to be a need to understand how symptoms progress and the effect on men and their partners. There is evidence showing that some symptoms do not resolve over time but rather become worse. This can interfere with quality of life and sense of normalcy. Providers play a crucial role in opening up the lines of communication, offering a safe environment for discussion, and providing treatment and referral if needed.

References

American Cancer Society. (1997). *Cancer source book for nurses*. Atlanta: Author.

Wein, A. J., Kavoussi, L. R., Novick, A. C., Partin, A. W., & Peters, G. A. (Eds.). (2009). *Campbell-Walsh urology*. Philadelphia: Elsevier.

Gailbraith, M. E., Pedro, L. W., Jaffe, A., & Allen, T. (2008). Describing health related outcomes for couples experiencing prostate cancer: Differences and similarities. *Oncology Nursing Forum 35*(5), 794–801.

⊗ FEMALE SEXUALITY

Laura Urquhart

A person's sexuality is a deeply personal issue. It is complex and incorporates multiple dimensions, which include physical, psychological, behavioral, and cultural aspects. The World Health Organization (WHO) defines sexuality as "the integration, somatic, emotional, intellectual and social aspects of sexual being that are positively enriching and enhance personality, communication and love" (WHO, 2002). Impairment in sexuality is a direct or indirect result of cancer treatment. Sexual dysfunction is the inability to express one's sexuality in a manner that is consistent with personal needs and preferences (Hughes, 1996). Common physical effects of cancer treatment are fatigue, nausea, skin changes, and menopause. Psychologically, the emotional impact of a cancer diagnosis and treatment tend to change the patient's primary focus to survival with sexual issues as a secondary issue.

Survivors may experience psychological distress related to altered body image as a temporary or permanent effect. Often, survivors relegate sexuality as a secondary need. The Lance Armstrong Foundation reports that 58% of cancer survivors deal with loss of sexual desire and/ or sexual function. Additionally, 33% of cancer survivors deal with infertility issues. The American Cancer Society (ACS) found that 64% of people with cancer had no sexual desire and that 48% had low sex drive after treatment with chemotherapy. Approximately 80% of women reported some change in sexual functioning up to 5 years after treatment for cancer. So, clearly, cancer diagnosis and treatment can affect intimacy and sexual functioning. The first step is assisting cancer survivors is validating their need for intimacy and sexual functioning despite age, gender, sexual orientation, religion, culture, and one's own life experiences. The next step of the assessment process is identifying treatment related factors, such as pain, body image changes, lost of desire, anxiety, depression, fear, guilt, and preexisting relationship issues.

In responding to survivors' sexual health needs it is important to understand the sexual cycle and how cancer treatment affects women's bodies and relationships. The sexual response cycle involves a sequence of biological and emotional events that occur in relation to sexual activity. The four components are desire (libido), arousal (excitement), orgasm, and resolution. Desire (libido) is an interest in sex, influenced by sight, touch, foreplay, and fantasies. For women, sexual desire also depends on emotional factors, including comfort level with sexuality, their partners, and feeling attractive. Testosterone and other hormones work in the brains of men and women to encourage sexual desire. Arousal occurs when the person's body reacts to stimulation by increasing the flow of blood to sexual organs. During the state of excitement, heart rate and blood pressure rise. In response to the excited state a woman's vagina will produce lubricant, and the walls will loosen and widen. The climax of pleasure is called orgasm. In both men and women, the nervous system creates intense pleasure in the genitals. The muscles around the genitals contract sending waves of feeling through the body. Men and women transition into the state of resolution a few minutes after climax with orgasm. The body becomes relaxed and the heart rate and blood pressure diminish. Blood drains out of the genitals and mental excitement subsides. Resolution is a period in which a person savors the encounter.

✺ Sexual Dysfunction

When a woman has difficulty with desire or arousal, her ability to reach satisfaction can be adversely affected. Additionally, a woman's sexual health and ability to be satisfied can be affected by her body image, self-esteem, identity, personal happiness, and the partner's actions, behaviors, and acceptance of her. Certainly, the impact of the diagnosis, even if an early stage disease, can make women feel vulnerable, angry, and frustrated.

There are two major factors that can greatly influence sexual function in women. First, the treatment itself can produce changes that affect sexual health, whether it's surgery, radiation, chemotherapy, or antiestrogen therapy. All of the preceding can trigger psychosocial issues such as altered body image and self-esteem, sense of loss, depression, anxiety, and changes in the relationship with the partner. Surgery may cause pain, affect mobility in the limbs, and disrupt lymph nodes and nerves. Some women suffer from neuropathic pain/hypersensitivity and negative body image as a long-term effect of treatments. Even women who choose reconstructive surgery suffer from the loss of tactile sensation and breast scarring (Bakewell & Volker, 2005). In regard to radiation, women will likely experience fatigue and skin reactions, during and immediately after treatment. Late effects of radiation may include skin pigmentation, skin thickening, retraction, and fibrosis (Horden, 2000). These can evolve over months to years after treatment.

Chemotherapy can adversely affect sexual health, producing many physical symptoms. Women may experience fatigue, malaise, nausea, vomiting, sleep disturbances, and gastrointestinal complaints; all can affect libido. One of the most recognizable side effects of chemotherapy is alopecia of the scalp and body hair, which can have a significant impact on a woman's body image and sense of physical attractiveness. Immunosuppression related to chemotherapy administration can trigger recurrence of genital herpes or genital warts in susceptible patients as well as put the woman at risk for developing vaginal yeast infections.

Last, there are vaginal symptoms related to chemotherapy-induced amenorrhea or menopause. Chemotherapy directly causes gonadal dysfunction through atresia of the ovarian stroma. The effect of chemotherapy on the ovarian stroma is age- and dose-dependent. Some younger women experience temporary amenorrhea, from which it may take up to 2 years to fully recover. Women who are 35 years and older are at the greatest risk for early menopause. The resulting loss of fertility can have enormous impact on the emotional and psychological health of women.

One other treatment that can affect sexual health is anti-estrogen therapy with selective estrogen receptor modulators (SERMs) or aromatase inhibitors (AIs). Selective estrogen receptor modulators, such as tamoxifen and raloxifene, act as an antagonist on many tissues in the body, producing many of the same side effects that are experienced during menopause, such as hot flashes/flushes and vaginal bleeding. Aromatase inhibitors such as letrozole, anastrozole, and exemestane work by inhibiting the production of estrogen in peripheral tissues and cancer tissue. In the peripheral tissues, male steroids are converted to estrogen by the aromatase enzyme. Aromatase inhibitors block the activity of this enzyme, resulting in a significant reduction of estrogen production. The mechanism of action leads to hot flashes and vaginal dryness through estrogen deprivation.

Women who experience early menopause and sexual side effects need to engage in a thorough and thoughtful discussion with their healthcare providers to evaluate the appropriateness of hormone replacement therapy. For those women diagnosed with breast cancer, regardless of estrogen receptor status, the use of topical or local estrogen treatment with creams, rings, or tablets is controversial and again a careful and thorough discussion should take place.

For those women who experience vaginal dryness possible treatments include lubricants that are water- or silicone-based, and vaginal moisturizing gels (Replens, K-Y liquid beads). The management of hot flashes first starts with education about lifestyle changes, such as dressing in layers and light clothing, lowering the room temperature, drinking cool beverages, and avoiding alcohol, warm beverages, and hot spicy foods. Pharmacologic treatment includes the use of antidepressants such as venlafaxine, paroxetine, citalopram, and sertraline. Other pharmacological agents used to treat hot flashes include antiepileptic agent gabapentin, clonidine, and vitamin E. Women taking 800 IU of vitamin E, an antioxidant largely composed of fat-soluble compounds (e.g., tocopherols), showed a reduction in hot flash symptoms that was equivalent to approximately one hot flash less per day than a placebo group (Sloan *et al.*, 2001). Other agents, such as black cohosh, soy-based preparations, and phytoestrogens, may have estrogenic activity (Boeckhout, Beijnen, & Schellens, 2006).

One of the most difficult tasks for oncology nurses may choose to undertake is to broach the subject of a survivor's sexual health. However, there can be benefits to starting such a conversation. It will show that it is a legitimate topic for discussion, and that providers treat the whole person (McKee & Shover, 2001). One of the most commonly used tools to assess sexuality is the Permission, Limited Information, Specific Suggestion, Intensive Therapy (PLISST) model (Annone, 1976). This model provides a framework for nursing assessment and care related to sexual health.

🕸 Summary

The causes of sexual dysfunction in cancer survivors is multifactorial. Sexual dysfunction is often viewed as a taboo subject. Oncology nurses can assist survivors by validating their concerns, assisting survivors with identification of causal factors, providing educational material, supplying information, and referrals to fertility specialists and sexual health counselors.

References

Annone, J. S. (1976). *The behavioral treatment of sexual problems: Brief therapy.* New York: Harper & Row.

Bakewell, R. T, & Volker, D. L. (2005). Sexual dysfunction related to treatment of young women with breast cancer. *Clinical Journal of Oncology Nursing, 9,* 697–702.

Boeckhout, A. H., Beijnen, J. H., & Schellens, J. H. (2006). Symptoms and treatment in cancer therapy-induced early menopause. *Oncologist, 11*(6), 641–654.

Horden, A. (2000). Intimacy and sexuality for women with breast cancer. *Cancer Nursing, 23*(3), 230–223.

Hughes, M. K. (1996). Sexuality issues: Keeping your cool. *Oncology Nursing Forum, 23,* 1597–1600.

McKee, A. L, & Schover, L. R. (2001). Sexuality rehabilitation. *Cancer, 92,* 1008–1012.

Sloan, J. A., Loprinzi, C. L., Novotny, P. J. Barton, D. L., Lavasseur, B. I., & Windshitl, H. (2001). Methodological lessons learned from hot flash studies. *Journal of Clinical Oncology, 19,* 4280–4290.

World Health Organization. (2002). Defining sexual health: a report of a technical consultation on sexual health. Accessed January 31, 2009, from http://www.who.int/reproductive-health/publications//sexualhealth/defining_sh.pdf

Bibliography

Ganz, P. A. (2007). *Cancer survivorship today and tomorrow.* New York: Springer.

Greendale, G. A., Petersen, L., & Zibecchi, L. (2001). Factors related to sexual function in post menopausal women with history of breast cancer. *Menopause, 8*(2), 111–119.

Hegel, M. T., Moore, C. L., Collins, E. D., Kearing, S., Gillock, K. L., Riggs, R. L., *et al.* (2006). Distress, psychiatric syndromes, and impairment of function in women with newly diagnosed breast cancer. *Cancer, 107,* 2924–2931.

Lance Armstrong Foundation: http://Livestrong.org

Love, S., & Lindsey, K. (1998). *Dr. Susan Love's Hormone Book. Making Informed Choices about Menopause.* New York: Three Rivers Press.

Mick, J. M. (2007). Sexuality assessment: 10 strategies for improvement. *Clinical Journal of Oncology Nursing*, *11*(5), 671–675.

Schover, L. R. (1997). *Sexuality and fertility after cancer.* New York: John Wiley and Sons.

Stilos, K., Doyle, C., & Daines, P. (2008). Addressing the sexual health needs of patients with gynecologic cancers. *Oncology Nursing Forum*, *12*(3), 457–463.

Wilmoth, M. C. (2006). Life after cancer: What does sexuality have to do with it? *Oncology Nursing Forum*, *33*(5), 905–910.

CHAPTER FIVE

Pharmacological Agents as Adjuvant Therapies

The treatment of lung cancer has improved the survival for many people facing this disease. With the advent of oral agents, many cancer survivors are caring for themselves at home rather than receiving intravenous chemotherapy infusions at outpatient oncology centers. Lung cancers may spread to the bone, requiring monthly intravenous infusions for bone metastases. This section will review adjuvant therapies for lung cancer, specifically those treatments that may continue for years after initial chemotherapy, surgery, and/or radiation therapy.

Oral Chemotherapy

The oral chemotherapeutic drug, erlotinib (Tarceva®), has been increasingly used to treat survivors with non-small-cell lung cancers who have failed one or more prior chemotherapy regimen(s). Erlotinib is a small molecule tyrosine kinase inhibitor (TKI) which inhibits activity of the epidermal growth factor receptor (EGFR). In 2004, the FDA approved for treatment of locally-advanced and metastatic non-small-cell lung cancers. To target TKI drugs such as erlotinib, sensitivity to the drug has been studied using tests to identify KRAS genetic mutations. The most common side effects of erlotinib are acneiform rash, diarrhea, paronychia, hypertrichosis, and, rarely, interstitial lung disease.

⑧ Bisphosphonates

For survivors who develop bone metastases, intravenous infusions of bisphosphonates may offer some protection from further boney erosion. The two most common types of bisphosphonates are zoledronic acid (Zometa®) and pamidronate (Aredia®). They both require intravenous infusion monthly and monitoring of electrolytes (calcium, magnesium, and phosphorus) as well as renal function (creatinine). Side effects include electrolyte abnormalities, compromised renal function, and osteonecrosis.

⑧ Bevacizumab

Ongoing infusion of antiangiogenesis agents such as bevacizumab (Avastin®) has been increasingly been integrated into first-line treatment for unresectable, non-small-cell lung cancers in conjunction with carboplatin and paclitaxel. Bevacizumab, monoclonal antibody, belongs to a class of antiangiogenesis drugs (i.e., drugs that block the formation and growth of new blood vessels by targeting a protein called vascular endothelial growth factor [VEGF]). Side effects include thromboembolic events.

⑧ New Drugs

Newer trials using drugs are ongoing and may provide evidence of increased efficacy in prolonging survival in cancer survivors with metastatic disease. Some new chemotherapy drugs, such as amrubicin, picoplatin, and sagopilone, are currently being tested in clinical trials.

Other drugs already approved for use against other types of cancer, such as sunitinib (Sutent®), thalidomide (Thalomid®), and sorafenib (Nexavar®), are now being tested for use against small cell lung cancer. Ongoing treatment may be part of survivorship care for people with advanced lung cancer requiring follow up with multiple healthcare providers on the oncology team and in the community. Communication between providers is essential to coordinating care and ensuring a comprehensive approach to the total person and not just the cancer. Oncology nurses are in a key position to help survivors address their concerns, teach about oral agents, monitor survivors at home, and coordinate care amongst multiple providers including visiting nurses, infusional services, physical therapy, and nutritional services.

Bibliography

National Cancer Institute. Clinical Trial Results (2009). Retrieved on February 11, 2009, from http://www.cancer.gov/clinicaltrials/

Sandler AB, Gray R, Brahmer J, et al. (2006). A randomized phase III trial of paclitaxel plus carboplatin with or without bevacizumab in patients with advanced non-squamous non-small cell lung cancer: An Eastern Cooperative Oncology Group Trial—E4599. *New England Journal of Medicine*, 355, 2542–2550.

CHAPTER SIX

Wellness and Healthy Behaviors

What is "normal?" This is the question that many people who have been diagnosed with cancer wonder after they complete treatment. Recovering from the initial treatment for cancer often requires healing from surgery, chemotherapy, and/or radiation treatments. It takes time to recover, and the first weeks after treatment may be filled with uncertainty as well as happiness. Survivors often look to life without treatment as a relief and sometimes as a time of worry. Ongoing monitoring by the oncology team provides a degree of security. Oncology nurses can support survivors as they transition to a lifestyle filled with fewer appointments as they resume self-care. As discussed in Chapter 3, ongoing follow-up and surveillance are useful in monitoring survivors for recurrence and side effects of treatment.

A diagnosis of cancer is often a time to reassess health and adopt a new, healthier lifestyle. It is a time to redefine health and create a "new normal," including healthier eating, more exercise, and even the addition of complementary therapies such as meditation and yoga. Oncology nurses play an important role in framing the "new normal" for survivors, stressing healthy living in all facets of life.

The National Comprehensive Cancer Network (2009) has published guidelines for survivorship care. These guidelines for follow-up are not just cancer-specific; they also address the basic principles of healthy lifestyles. Included in the NCCN Guidelines are recommendations for:

- Maintaining a healthy weight
- Encouraging a physically active lifestyle
- Screening and counseling for alcohol and tobacco use
- Counseling regarding healthy eating with an emphasis on plant sources

Routine health monitoring should be maintained or resumed by all cancer survivors. Examples of routine health monitoring and screening include:

- Measurement of blood pressure, cholesterol, and glucose levels
- Bone density testing (if appropriate)
- Routine dental care
- Sun protection
- Vaccinations for pneumococcus and influenza annually as well as herpes zoster
- Screening for depression

The overall care for most cancer survivors is coordinated between the oncology team and the primary care provider (see Chapter 9 for more on Coordination of Care). In this section, the principles of survivorship care are reviewed, including healthy behaviors focused on wellness. Some guidelines and preventive behaviors are disease-specific, whereas others integrate principles of health promotion with screening guidelines.

The following topics are covered in this chapter:

- Nutrition
- Exercise
- Smoking cessation
- Complementary therapies
- Bone health

⊗ NUTRITION
Jeannine Mills

⊗ Introduction

Early and intensive nutrition intervention is beneficial in minimizing weight loss, deterioration in nutritional status, global quality of life, and physical function in cancer patients (Ravasco, Monteiro Grillo, & Camilo, 2003; Ravasco, Monteiro-Grillo, Vidal, & Camilo, 2005a,b). Cancer patients must meet calorie and protein needs to prevent weight loss, preserve lean body mass, and maintain protein stores. Weight loss as a result of treatment or therapy can result in the loss of protein and fat stores for energy contributing to muscle wasting and fatigue. Fifteen to forty percent of all patients with solid tumors experience weight loss at diagnosis. Sixty percent of patients with lung cancer experience weight loss and 80% of patients with upper gastrointestinal cancers experience weight loss at diagnosis (Centers for Disease Control and Prevention, 2009). Reversible weight loss may occur when patients experience starvation or malnutrition secondary to side effects experienced from chemotherapy, radiation therapy, or surgery. In reversible weight loss, lean body mass is typically preserved by a greater loss in fat mass and only a mild negative nitrogen balance may occur. In tumor-induced weight loss or cancer cachexia, weight loss is characterized by muscle wasting, anorexia, asthenia, depression, and chronic nausea. As opposed to reversible weight loss, cancer cachexia is very difficult to reverse. There is a loss of lean body mass and fat mass, muscle wasting, significant negative nitrogen balance, metabolic derangements, and neuroendocrine alterations. Factors involved in both reversible weight loss and cancer cachexia may occur at any time in the cancer care continuum.

Sixty percent of cancer patients experience some form of malnutrition during cancer treatment, which includes surgery, chemotherapy, and radiation therapy. In addition, posttreatment challenges can continue to additionally burden a compromised nutritional status. Postsurgical patients must increase energy and nutrient requirements with the demands of wound healing. Patients undergoing chemotherapy may experience anemia, fatigue, nausea, vomiting, diarrhea, dysgeusia (altered taste), and depression. Radiation therapy can deplete calorie intake and nutrient stores secondary to diarrhea, fistula formations, dysphagia (difficulty swallowing) for solids and/or liquids, mucositis, and esophagitis.

⊛ Assessment

Meeting the challenge by providing optimal nutritional therapy requires regular screening and assessment of cancer survivors during and after therapy. Survivors are at high nutritional risk if their weight loss exceeds 2.5% in 1 week, 5% in 1 month, or 10% in 6 months. Other indicators of malnutrition include body mass index (BMI) less than 17 kg/m^2, prealbumin less than 15 mg/dl, and serum albumin less than 3.5 mg/dl (Elliot, Molseed, McCallum, & Grant, 2006).

The benefits of nutrition interventions include improvement of immune function, better tolerance to treatment, improved healing and recovery times, improved strength and endurance, and a sense of well-being. Baseline screening identifies nutritional risk and repeated assessments identify those who require intervention. The Nutrition Care Process was instituted by American Dietetic Association in 2002 and provides the framework to provide nutritional care, including nutrition assessment, nutrition diagnosis, nutrition intervention, and nutrition monitoring and evaluation (Lacey & Pritchett, 2003). Several nutrition screening and assessment tools are available to nurses, but ideally the tool should be one that is simple to use, validated, and includes a plan of care.

Faith Ottery designed the Scored Patient-Generated Subjective Global Assessment to meet the needs of the oncology population (Bauer, Capra, & Ferguson, 2003). This validated tool scores common nutrition impact symptoms, degree of weight loss, metabolic demands, and physical exam in order to determine nutritional risk and level of intervention. Many institutions have adapted abridged versions; however, any adaptation should also undergo validation.

Interventions

Nurses can be the first to identify and recommend nutritional strategies to manage side effects from treatment. Altered taste or dysgeusia can occur in greater than 50% of cancer survivors. Review of oral care can be effective as dysgeusia can be a result of dry mouth, fungal infections, and poor oral care. Some survivors can taste but to a much lesser degree, which is referred to as hypogeusia. Strategies to manage altered taste include eating moist foods, being creative in seasoning foods with fresh herbs and lemon, marinate meats, and choosing fresh as opposed to canned or frozen produce.

Poor appetite can be a result of pain, constipation, nausea, or depression. Working with the survivor and care providers to identify the source of the complaints can allow better management of the problem. Encourage eating every 2 hours with small, calorie-dense meals. Avoid skipping meals if possible. Suggest that care providers provide gentle encouragement. Create a dining atmosphere that is quiet, comfortable, and relaxing. Various appetite stimulants can be recommended, including dronabinol, megestrol acetate, corticosteroids, anabolic agents, and metoclopramide.

Constipation, a frequent cause of diminished appetite, may be attributed to decreased activity, decreased food and fluid intake, pain and opioid use, fatigue, and medication (antidepressants), or may be chemotherapy-induced. Bowel regimens are warranted for any patient taking narcotics. Laxatives may include stool softeners, stimulants, bulk-forming agents, hyperosmotic laxatives, lubricants, saline laxatives, and osmotic cathartics. Nutritional management of constipation first considers if the person is meeting fluid needs. Increasing fiber-rich foods in the diet may be helpful in regulating bowels. Bulk-forming agents such as psyllium must be taken with adequate fluid. These agents are not recommended for anyone who has poor mobility or is at risk for bowel obstruction. Side effects may include bloating, gas, cramping, and distention. When constipation is a problem, talk about limiting gas-forming foods and carbonated beverages, using drinking straws, or chewing gum, all of which can increase gas.

Diarrhea may affect nutritional status and hydration and may be caused by multiple factors. Chemotherapy may irritate the gastrointestinal tract, causing frequent loose stools. Radiation therapy may decrease the absorptive capacity of the gastrointestinal tract. Diarrhea may be exacerbated by high-fat foods, high caffeine, simple sugars, high-fiber foods including fresh fruits and vegetables, as well as gas-producing foods. Patients receiving treatment should be instructed to drink 8 ounces of fluid for every loose bowel movement. Repletion of potassium and sodium also should be recommended with foods high in both. Soluble forms of fiber, such as oat bran, banana, applesauce, and barley help to bulk the stool.

Lactose intolerance may also develop in some patients undergoing radiation therapy or after such surgeries as Whipple resection or esophagectomy. Some patients may find that simply reducing dairy products to no more than 2 cups a day may be helpful, whereas others may need to switch entirely to lactose-free products.

Esophagitis can be a result of radiation therapy, as seen in lung cancer and esophageal cancer therapies. A soft, bland, semiliquid diet may be recommended. Foods that are tart, coarse, acidic, or salty can add to the discomfort of swallowing. Lukewarm or cool foods are tolerated best. Alcohol, tobacco, and caffeine can all exacerbate soreness with swallowing. Some patients find weak tea or tea with honey soothing to swallow.

Mucositis can be a complication of both radiation therapy and chemotherapy. It is an inflammation of the mucosal cells of the gastrointestinal tract, and can decrease absorption of nutrients. Mouth care is essential, including general good hygiene, topical anesthetics, antifungal agents if necessary, and systemic analgesics. Attention to dietary alterations is also recommended. Foods that are soft, moist, and low in acidity are generally better tolerated. Carbonated beverages and extreme temperatures in liquids and solids can also be irritants to the mucosa. Encourage people with dentures to only wear them when eating or not at all. Take the time to examine the oral mucosa for signs of oral candidiasis, a common infectious cause of mucositis.

Dry mouth or xerostomia as well as increased phlegm can be most problematic among head/neck cancer patients receiving radiation therapy as part of their treatment plan. Hydration is imperative in this population. Again, oral care is essential, as these patients may be more susceptible to mouth infections. To stimulate flow of saliva, encourage patients to suck on lemon drops or chew sugarless gum. Some patients find it helpful to rinse the mouth with seltzer, ginger ale, or club soda and lemon juice. Pineapple or papaya juice have been found to be useful in relieving thick phlegm because of the natural enzymes in both fruits. Dry mouth sprays are commercially available and offer temporary relief. Patients can make their own dry mouth spray with a few drops of glycerin added to a small spray bottle of water. Alcohol and caffeine may also contribute to dry mouth and should be limited if possible.

Chemotherapy-induced nausea and vomiting (CINV) is considered among the most significant adverse events after therapy. It may significantly hamper a survivor's ability to perform daily activities, including preparing and enjoying meals. First and foremost, nausea should be treated with an antiemetic protocol. Nutritional recommendations include reviewing fluid needs, recommending small frequent meals, avoiding foods with strong odors, consuming foods that are cool or room temperature, avoiding overly sweet or fried foods, and rinsing the mouth before and after meals. Ginger or peppermint tea may also be helpful.

⑧ Nutrition in Survivorship

There are more than 24 million cancer survivors worldwide, with 12 million in the United States alone. Breast, colorectal, and prostate cancers make up 50% of the total number of survivors (Institute of Medicine, 2005). It has been said that a "cancer diagnosis is a teachable moment," and we see that many cancer survivors want to initiate diet changes after diagnosis. In a study looking at 354 Finnish and Australian breast cancer patients after diagnosis (Salminen, Bishop, Poussa, Drummond, & Salminen, 2004), 30–39% of women made diet changes on their own initiative. This study suggested that there is a high need for dietary counseling, and this need is unrecognized by their healthcare providers. A landmark study known as the Women's Intervention Nutrition Study (WINS) was a Phase III study that examined dietary fat restriction in postmenopausal women with primary breast cancer (Chlebowski et al., 2005). The study considered whether a 15–20% fat diet would reduce recurrence risk. The results showed a 9.8% recurrence with a low-fat diet, versus a 12.4% recurrence with a normal diet. The lead investigator commented that "this is a strong signal that breast cancer patients can reduce risk of recurrence by lowering the amount of dietary fat they consume." With breast cancer, studies suggest an increased risk of mortality from early-stage breast cancer associated with women who are obese or overweight at diagnosis and after treatment. Normal, overweight, and obese survivors should be advised to avoid weight gain during cancer treatments. Weight loss may be safe and possibly helpful in overweight and obese cancer survivors who are otherwise healthy (Rock & Denmark-Wahnefried, 2002).

Cancer survivors also have to confront late and/or lingering effects of therapy, including congestive heart failure, osteoporosis, neuropathy, premature menopause, diarrhea, and weight gain/weight loss. The evidence is overwhelming that cancer survivors may die from noncancer causes at a higher rate than the general population such as diabetes, hypertension, and cardiovascular disease. The Institute of Medicine (2005) has suggested a Survivorship Care Plan that includes nutritional guidelines for cancer survivors.

1. Choose predominantly plant-based diets rich in variety of fruits and vegetables.
2. If eaten at all, limit red meat to less than 3 ounces daily.
3. Limit consumption of fatty foods, particularly those of animal origin. Choose modest amounts of appropriate vegetable oils.
4. Limit consumption of salted foods and use of cooking oil and table salt. Use herbs and spices to season foods.
5. Limit alcoholic drinks to less than two drinks a day for men and one for women.
6. Do not eat charred food. Consume the following only occasionally: meat and fish grilled in direct flame, and cured and smoked meats.
7. Avoid being overweight and limit weight gain during adulthood. Take an hour's brisk walk or similar exercise daily.

The American Cancer Society (ACS) published recommendations in their report, *Nutrition and Physical Activity During and After Cancer Treatment: An American Cancer Society Guide for Informed Choices* (Doyle *et al.*, 2006). They state that "although scientific evidence for advice on nutrition and physical activity after cancer is much less certain than for cancer prevention, it is likely that following the ACS guidelines on diet, nutrition and cancer prevention may be helpful for reducing the risk of developing secondary cancers." These guidelines are also in line with recommendations for prevention of cardiovascular disease, diabetes, and osteoporosis.

American Cancer Society Guidelines on Nutrition and Physical Activity for Cancer Prevention include:

1. Maintain a healthy weight throughout life.
    a. Balance a caloric intake with physical activity.
    b. Avoid excessive weight gain throughout the life cycle.
    c. Achieve and maintain a healthy weight if currently overweight or obese.

2. Adopt a physically active lifestyle.
    a. Adults: engage in at least 30 minutes of moderate-to-vigorous physical activity, above usual activities, on 5 or more days of the week. Forty-five to 60 minutes of intentional physical activity are preferable.
    b. Children and adolescents: engage in at least 60 minutes per day of moderate-to-vigorous physical activity at least 5 days a week.

3. Consume a healthy diet, with an emphasis on plant-based foods.
    a. Choose foods and beverages in amounts that help achieve and maintain a healthy weight.
    b. Eat five or more servings of a variety of vegetables and fruits each day.

   c. Choose whole grains in preference to processed (refined) grains.

   d. Limit consumption of processed red meats.

4. If you drink alcoholic beverages, limit consumption.

   a. Drink no more than one drink per day for women or two per day for men.

Vitamin and supplement use is common among the 12 million cancer survivors in the United States. A recent review on the topic found "in studies combining different cancer sites, 64–81% of survivors reported using any vitamin or mineral supplements and 26–77% reported using any multivitamins" (Velicer & Ulrich, 2008). Breast cancer survivors reported the highest use of vitamins and supplements. Also, higher level of education and female sex were consistently associated with supplement use. The review concludes the uncertainty of harm or benefit with multivitamin use among cancer patients or long-term survivors, and if benefit or harm varies according to before, during, or after treatment. Healthcare providers should be cautious when counseling survivors about supplement use, as there are some vitamins and minerals that may actually be involved in cancer progression after the carcinogenic process has been initiated. There is also concern that some supplements may interact with cancer treatments by decreasing effectiveness of treatment by blocking reactive oxygen species. Other studies show improvement in nutritional status among supplement users who had an otherwise poor diet. Some studies also show an improvement in survival in those who reported using vitamins and mineral supplements.

🕮 Summary

Clinical dietitians are an integral part of the healthcare team in the oncology setting. As of 2008, oncology dietitians can now take an examination through the Center of Dietetic Registration to become Board Certified Specialists in Oncology. Contact the American Dietetic Association to locate a clinical dietitian in your state or community.

References

Bauer, J., Capra, S., & Ferguson, M. (2003). Use of the scored Patient-Generated Subjective Global Assessment and its association with quality of life in ambulatory patients receiving radiotherapy. *European Journal of Clinical Nutrition, 57,* 305–309.

Centers for Disease Control and Prevention. Retrieved on February 16, 2009, from, http://www.cdc.gov/

Chlebowski, R. T., Blackburn, G. L., Elashoff, R. E., *et al.* (2005). Dietary fat reduction in postmenopausal women with primary breast cancer: Phase III Women's Intervention Nutrition Study (WINS). *Proceedings of the American Society of Clinical Oncology, 23,* 3.

Doyle, C., Kushi, L. H., Byer, T., Courneya, K. S., Demark-Wahnefried, W., Grant, B., *et al.* (2006). Nutrition and physical activity during and after cancer treatment: An American Cancer Society guide for informed choices. *Cancer, 56,* 323–353.

Elliot, L., Molseed, L., McCallum, P. D., & Grant, B., (Eds.) (2006). *The clinical guide to oncology nutrition.* Chicago: American Dietetic Association.

Institute of Medicine. (2005). *From cancer patient to cancer survivor: Lost in transition.* Washington, DC: Institute of Medicine of the National Academies.

Lacey, K., & Pritchett, E. (2003). Nutrition care process and model: ADA adopts road map to quality care and outcomes. *Journal of the American Dietetic Association, 103,* 1061–1072.

Ravasco, P., Monteiro-Grillo, I., & Camilo, M. E. (2003). Does nutrition influence quality of life in cancer patients undergoing radiotherapy? *Radiotherapeutic Oncology, 67*(2), 213–220.

Ravasco, P., Monteiro-Grillo, I., Vidal, P. M., & Camilo, M. E. (2005a). Dietary counseling improves patient outcomes: A prospective, randomized, controlled trial in colorectal cancer patients undergoing radiotherapy. *Journal of Clinical Oncology, 23*(7), 1431–1438.

Ravasco, P., Monteiro-Grillo, I., Vidal, P. M., & Camilo, M. E. (2005b). Impact of nutrition on outcome: A prospective randomized controlled trial in patients with head and neck cancer undergoing radiotherapy. *Head and Neck, 27*(8), 659–668.

Rock, C. L., & Denmark-Wahnefried, W. (2002). Can lifestyle modification increase survival in woman diagnosed with breast cancer? *Journal of Nutrition, 132,* 3540s–35409s.

Salminen, E., Bishop, M., Poussa, T., Drummond, R., & Salminen, S. (2004). Dietary attitudes and changes as well as use of supplements and complementary therapies by Australian and Finnish women following the diagnosis of breast cancer. *European Journal of Clinical Nutrition, 58*(1), 137–144.

Velicer, C., & Ulrich, C. M. (2008). Vitamin and mineral supplement use among US adults after cancer diagnosis: A systemic review. *Journal of Clinical Oncology, 26,* 665–673.

Bibliography

Eldridge, B., & Hamilton, K. (2003). Management of nutrition impact symptoms in cancer and educational handouts. *Journal of the American Dietetic Association, 107*(3), 412–415.

Ottery, F. D. (1995). Supportive nutrition to prevent cachexia and improve quality of life. *Seminars in Oncology, 22,* 98–111.

Web Sites

American Cancer Society: http://www.cancer.org

American Dietetic Association: http://www.eatright.org

American Institute for Cancer Research: http://www.aicr.org

Caring for Cancer: http://www.caring4cancer.com

Diana Dyer: http://www.CancerRD.com

National Coalition of Cancer Survivorship: http://www.canceradvocacy.org

Oncolink: http://www.oncolink.upenn.edu

Oncology Nutrition Dietetic Practice Group: http://www.oncologynutrition.org

Pancreatic Cancer Action Network: http://www.pancan.org

Excellent resources for dietary supplements include the following Web sites:

Center for Complementary and Alternative Medicine (NCCAM): http://nccam.nih.gov

http://www.Consumerlab.com

http://www.Naturaldatabase.com

http://www.Micromedix.com

Office of Dietary Supplements: http://ods.od.nih.gov/

Stephen Barrett's Quack Watch: http://www.quackwatch.org

EXERCISE

Charlene Gates

Introduction

Exercise has been shown to have many benefits for people with cancer. Surgery, radiation, and chemo/hormonal therapy have acute and long-term effects that can be positively affected by physical activity. Survivors often decrease their activity level for months or years after treatment ends. This may also be caused by side effects of treatment, negative affect, or perceived barriers to exercise. Decreases in physical activity result in further losses of strength and endurance, which then exacerbate fatigue levels. Nurses can encourage survivors to interrupt this cycle by staying active and helping them to understand that exercise can counteract the physical, functional, psychological, and emotional effects of cancer treatment. Education regarding the benefits of physical activity should be a part of inpatient support, postoperative instructions, chemotherapy teaching, and continue during posttreatment visits. Referral to physical therapy is beneficial to address specific deficits or provide guidance and support to get started with an exercise program.

The majority of the research on the effects of physical activity has been devoted to cancer prevention or the effects during treatment. Physical activity can have positive effects on both the acute and late or long-term results of cancer treatment. Late effects are caused by complications that are absent or subclinical when treatment is completed, but emerge much later as significant problems that can be attributed to the effects of treatment. An example is development of an arrhythmia several years after treatment with a cardiotoxic chemotherapy drug (e.g., doxorubican). A long-term effect is a side effect that appears during or immediately after treatment and persists for months or years. Table 6-1 summarizes the late and long-term effects of cancer treatment that may be positively affected by physical activity.

TABLE 6-1   Late and Long-Term Effects of Cancer Treatment That May Be Positively Affected by Physical Activity

---

Cancer Treatments: Surgery, Radiation, Chemotherapy, Immunotherapy, Hormone Therapy, Steroid Therapy

Physical Changes:

- Pulmonary function
- Cardiac function
- Muscle mass
- Fat mass
- Weight or BMI
- Decreased muscle strength/power
- Inflammation
- Immune function
- Bone health
- Trauma and scarring
- Lymphatic function (lymphedema)

Psychological and Behavioral Changes:

- Exercise/physical activity
- Physical symptoms and pain
- Depression
- Cognitive function
- Quality of life (multiple domains)

⚛ Contraindications to Exercise

There have been many myths about exercise for people with cancer. These include worsening cardiotoxicity from chemotherapy or radiation therapy, suppressing the immune system, exaggerating nausea or fatigue, and causing pathologic bone fractures by stressing bone compromised by metastatic disease. These fears have not been confirmed by research or experience. There have been no significant adverse events reported in studies of exercise interventions with cancer patients. However, there are important conditions in which exercise is contraindicated or caution is needed. Currently accepted contraindications and precautions are given in Table 6-2.

TABLE 6-2   Contraindications and Precautions During Treatment and Afterward

Contraindication	Comment
Complete blood counts	Hemoglobin level <8.0 g/dl Avoid activities that require significant oxygen transports (i.e., high intensity)
Absolute neutrophil count ≤500	Avoid activities that may increase risk of bacterial infection (e.g., swimming)
Platelet count <50,000	Avoid activities that increase risk of bleeding (e.g., contact sports, high-impact exercises)
Fever greater than 38°C (100.4°F)	May indicate system infection and should be investigated; avoid high-intensity exercise

TABLE 6-2 (continued)

Ataxia, dizziness, or peripheral sensory neuropathy	Avoid activities that require significant balance and coordination (e.g., tread-mill exercise)
Severe cachexia (loss of > 35% of premorbid weight)	Loss of muscle mass usually limits exercise to mild intensity, depending on degree of cachexia
Dyspnea	Investigate cause; exercise to tolerance
Bone pain	Avoid activities that increase risk of fracture (e.g., contact sports, high impact exercises)
Severe nausea	Investigate cause; exercise to tolerance
Extreme fatigue and/or muscle weakness	Exercise to tolerance

From: Courneya, Mackey, & Jones, 2000.

Summary of Benefits of Exercise for Cancer Survivors

1. *Acute physiologic outcomes and symptom/side effects.* There is consistent evidence for a positive effect of physical activity interventions on physiologic outcomes, symptoms/side effects, and immune variables for patients during active treatment. The physiologic outcomes included in these studies included blood and platelet transfusions, body temperature, in-hospital days, and loss of physical function during hospitalization (Schmitz *et al.*, 2005). The patient groups that have been studied are primarily those receiving high-dose chemotherapy and bone marrow transplants.

2. *Cardiorespiratory fitness.* Several of the chemotherapy drugs potentially have cardiotoxic effects. In addition, radiation to the chest can also cause some damage to cardiac muscle or lung tissue, although the risk is less with modern tangential techniques. Numerous randomized controlled trials of various exercise interventions of moderate intensity for cancer survivors have all shown positive effects.

3. *Muscular strength and endurance.* Several studies with breast cancer survivors utilizing resistance training, tai chi, or yoga have all shown a positive effect. Most recently, an observational study of 132 cancer survivors with a variety of diagnoses participating in a gym-based resistive exercise program showed significant improvements in both upper and lower extremity strength. This was one of the few studies that included survivors with stage IV disease (Litterini & Fieler, 2008).

4. *Flexibility.* Surgery and radiation can result in limitations of flexibility and range of motion (ROM). Active movement and stretching exercises at the appropriate stage of recovery can reverse these limitations. Most of the studies on flexibility have been done with breast cancer patients. Tai chi, dance, or aerobic exercise and stretching have all been shown to improve shoulder ROM in these patients (Physical Activity Guidelines Advisory Committee Report, 2008).

5. *Weight change and body composition.* Exercise has a potential impact on undesirable changes in body composition. For some cancers (non-small cell lung, pancreatic, renal cell, and head/neck cancer), systemic inflammation may contribute to loss of lean body mass (Silver, Dietrich, & Murphy, 2007). For these diagnoses, preserving muscle is a priority. For breast cancer, overall weight gain and increased ratio of adipose tissue to lean body

mass is an unwanted effect of adjuvant chemotherapy and hormonal therapy. Physical activity can preserve muscle mass and also contribute to decreased risk of weight gain. However, it will likely have little to no effect if calories are not restricted (Physical Activity Guidelines Advisory Committee Report, 2008).

6. *Mental health/quality of life.* Studies on exercise after a cancer diagnosis have consistently shown a positive effect in many domains of quality of life, including physical, functional, social, and emotional well-being (Courneya *et al.*, 2000). These studies have focused on patients undergoing bone marrow transplants or survivors of breast, colorectal, or prostate cancer. They have demonstrated positive results for patients who participate in an exercise program during treatment, whether supervised or a home-based program. Outcome measures show improved life satisfaction, quality of life, depression, anxiety, mood, coping behaviors, cancer-related symptoms, physical performance, and fatigue.

7. *Fatigue levels.* Persistent fatigue affects the majority of cancer survivors. It interferes with activities of daily living and is more prevalent than pain. Research has shown that decreased exercise performance capacity is significantly correlated with fatigue for cancer patients completing chemotherapy and bone marrow transplantation. However, fatigue is a multidimensional problem thought to be caused by physical, psychological, and other diverse factors (Stricker, Drake, Hoyer, & Mock, 2004). Moderate aerobic exercise has successfully been used as a strategy for managing fatigue. Exercise interventions utilizing a stationary bike, treadmill walking, or supervised walking programs at home have all shown correlations with decreased fatigue, primarily with breast cancer patients.

8. *Decreased risk of recurrence and mortality.* Research in the last few years has also demonstrated that survivors of stage I to III breast cancer who include moderate physical activity (approximately 4–5 weekly 30-minute sessions of brisk walking) improve their survival rate from breast cancer and overall mortality from other causes by 50–60% compared with less active survivors. Obesity and weight gain are associated with breast cancer recurrence. In two studies on survivors of colorectal cancer, there were similar findings, although the level of activity to achieve the effect was higher (Physical Activity Guidelines Advisory Committee Report, 2008).

🎗 Current Exercise Guidelines

Guidelines for Physical Activity were announced by the US Department of Health and Human Services (HHS) in 2008 and are similar for early-stage cancer patients, cancer survivors, and the general population. The report that accompanied the announcement of the guidelines includes a chapter summarizing the research on physical activity for individuals who have been treated for cancer. The panel of experts convened by HHS concluded that most health benefits occur with at least 2.5 hours (150 minutes) a week of moderate-intensity physical activity, such as brisk walking. Additional benefits occur with more physical activity. Episodes of activity that are at least 10 minutes long count toward meeting the Guidelines. Frequency should be three to five times per week, or daily for patients who are deconditioned and are doing light-intensity, shorter-duration periods of exercise. Intensity should be moderate (perceived exertion, or 50–75% vO_2max or HR reserve). Frequency and duration goals should be met before increasing intensity. Although there is less evidence, strength training is recommended two to three times per week.

The exercise prescription should be modified based on baseline fitness level, musculoskeletal impairments, comorbid conditions, and chemotherapy cycles. Safety is critical. Patients with central venous access catheters, catheters, urostomies, colostomies, or cancer affecting bone need special consideration. In the past, women were advised to avoid exercise after having axillary node dissections for breast cancer. Research over the past several years has shown no increased risk of developing lymphedema, or exacerbation of lymphedema in patients who have this condition.

Steps for Patients Starting an Exercise Program

1. *Assess fitness level*. Resting heart rate (HR) body-mass index (BMI = height to weight ratio), waist circumference, or distance walking comfortably in 10 minutes

2. *Design an exercise program*. Take into account preferences, daily routine, and any limitations (e.g., neuropathy affecting balance)

3. *Get equipment ready*. Calendar, shoes, appropriate clothing, pedometer, watch

4. *Get started*. Increase gradually and adjust for the survivor's tolerance and response, following the recommendations to increase duration and frequency before increasing intensity, and record progress!

5. *Keep track of progress*. Check the resting HR and BMI.

Strategies for Success

1. Write it down! It is very rewarding to see progress and it is an important behavioral tool.

2. Use visual cues such as leaving walking shoes or exercise clothing by the door.

3. Plan ahead and schedule exercise time, making it part of a routine.

4. Enlist the company and support of friends or family.

5. Plan rewards for reaching milestones!

❧ Summary

It's important to remember that many people have no symptoms when they are diagnosed with cancer. Their goal is to return to the life they had before treatment and put cancer in their past. Some survivors use their cancer experience as a basis for making lifestyle changes. Nurses are ideally positioned to support people with cancer during treatment by emphasizing the role of exercise in maintaining strength. They can also help cancer survivors by including exercise as part of their recovery and survivorship plan to develop a healthy lifestyle in survivorship.

References

Courneya, K. S., & Freidenreich, C. M. (2001). Framework PEACE: an organizational model for examining physical exercise across the cancer experience. *Annals of Behavioral Medicine, 23,* 263–72.

Courneya, K. S., Mackey, J. R., & Jones, L. W. (2000). Coping with cancer: can exercise help? *The Physician and Sportsmedicine, 28*(5), 49–51, 55–66, 66–68, 71–73.

Litterini, A. J., & Fieler, V. K. (2008). The change in fatigue, strength, and quality of life following a physical therapist prescribed exercise program for cancer survivors. *Rehabilitation Oncology, 26*(3), 11–17.

Schmitz, K. H., Holtzman, J., Courneya, K. S., Masse, L. C., Duval, S., & Kane, R. (2005). Controlled physical activity trials in cancer survivors: a systematic review and meta-analysis. *Cancer Epidemiological Biomarkers Preview, 14*(7), 1588–1595.

Stricker, C. T., Drake, D., Hoyer, K., & Mock, V. (2004). Evidence-based practice for fatigue management in adults with cancer: exercise as an intervention. *Oncology Nursing Forum, 31*(5), 963–976.

Bibliography

Doyle, C., Kushi, I.. H., Byers, T., Courneya, K. S., Mark-Wahnefried, W., Grant, B., *et al*. (2006). Nutrition and physical activity during and after cancer treatment: An American Cancer Society guide for informed choices. *Cancer Journal for Clinicians, 56*(6), 323–353.

Silvei, H. J., Dietrich, M. S., & Murphy, B. A. (2007). Changes in body mass, energy balance, physical function, and inflammatory state in patients with locally advanced head and neck cancer treated with concurrent chemoradiation after low-dose induction chemotherapy. *Head Neck, 29*(10), 893–900.

Web Sites

2008 Physical Guidelines for Americans and 2008 Physical Activity Guidelines Advisory Committee Report. U.S. Department of Health and Human Services. Retrieved on February 2, 2009 from www.health.gov/PAGuidelines/Default.aspx

BMI Calculator. Retrieved on February 2, 2009 from www.mayoclinic.com

Exercise May Improve Survival & Exercise for Fatigue. Retrieved on February 2, 2009, from www.breastcancer.org

SMOKING CESSATION/TOBACCO TREATMENT

Wendye DiSalvo

Introduction

The World Health Organization (WHO) estimates there are 1.3 billion smokers globally, with an estimated tobacco related mortality of 10 million deaths by 2030. In the United States, there are 45 million adult cigarette smokers, with 435,000 tobacco-related deaths annually. The sequela of tobacco use accounts for serious illness in 8.6 million Americans per year. Because of this significant morbidity and mortality, treatment of tobacco addiction is paramount (WHO, 2008). In addition, nearly one third of all cancers are caused by smoking. Despite this statistic, it has been estimated that 20% of cancer survivors continue to smoke because of fatalistic attitudes that it is too late to quit. On the contrary, cessation of tobacco use has been associated with improved tolerance to treatment, improved survival, and a decreased risk of developing a secondary cancer (Gritz, 2006).

Individuals who quit smoking reduce the risk of premature death by 50% within 5 years of cessation, and the risk of premature death is nearly identical to lifelong nonsmokers within 15 years. The risk of developing lung cancer in smokers is 20 times higher for men and 12 times higher for women than it is for nonsmokers. There is a 30–50% decreased risk of lung cancer after 10 years of abstinence. The longer the cessation, the greater the risk reduction. The risk of developing cancer of the oral cavity is 20 times higher in male smokers and 5–10 times greater in female smokers. Quitting reduces the risk by 50% as soon as 5 years of abstinence. The risk of developing esophageal cancer is 5–10 times higher in smokers, but with cessation the risk is reduced by 50% in 5 years. The risk of developing pancreatic cancer is 2–3 times higher in smokers, but the effects of smoking cessation are measured after 10 years of abstinence. Both men and women smokers have a 2–4 times higher risk of developing bladder cancer, but after only a few years the risk is reduced by 50%. Women who smoke have a 2–3 times higher risk of developing cervical cancer, and cessation sustainably reduces risk even after a few years. Other comorbid conditions that have risk reduction after smoking cessation include coronary heart disease (CHD), peripheral artery occlusive disease, ischemic strokes and subarachnoid hemorrhage, respiratory symptoms, chronic obstructive lung disease (COPD) and COPD mortality, low birth weight infants, early onset of menopause, and duodenal and gastric ulcers (Abrams *et al.*, 2003).

As oncology nurses, it is imperative to understand the basics of tobacco addiction and why it is so difficult for smokers to quit. Addiction is characterized by compulsive drug seeking and use, even though there are significant health consequences (National Institute of Drug Abuse Tobacco Addiction, 2009). More than 4000 chemicals are found in tobacco smoke. The chemical directly involved in addiction is nicotine. On average, the smoker receives 1–2 mg of nicotine per cigarette. Snuff and chew also contain nicotine. Those individuals who use pipes and cigars absorb nicotine through mucosal membranes (Federal Trade Commission, 2000). Nicotine stimulates the adrenal glands to release adrenaline with a resultant "kick." The release of adrenaline causes a sudden release of glucose and increases heart rate, blood pressure, and respiration (Benowitz, 1996). Nicotine activates the reward pathway of the brain, which is associated with the feelings of pleasure. Nicotine binds to nicotinic acetylcholine receptors in the brain; the primary receptor is the a4B2 nicotinic receptor in the ventral tegmental area (VTA). This results in the release of the neurotransmitter dopamine in the nucleus accumbens, which is believed to be linked to reward. Within 10 seconds of inhalation there is rapid distribution of nicotine to the brain. The acute effects of nicotine dissipate within a few minutes as well as the feeling of reward. Thus, the smoker seeks to maintain the drug's pleasurable effects and avoid withdrawal (Benowitz, 1996).

Nicotine withdrawal syndrome is seen as a true sign of dependence. The syndrome includes irritability, frustration, anger, anxiety, restlessness, decreased heart rate, craving, cognitive and attentional deficits, insomnia, and increased appetite (Hughes & Hatsukami, 1992). Withdrawal can start as soon as 2 hours after the last use of tobacco, and often peaks 24–48 hours after cessation. The symptoms can last for days to months (Piasecki, Fiore, & Baker, 1997).

Assessing a smoker's readiness to quit is imperative. Approximately 90% of smokers say they want to quit smoking, but 70% are not ready to quit in the next 6 months, and fewer than 20% are willing to quit in the next month (Velicer *et al.*, 1995). The use of The Stages of Change or Transtheoretical Model can guide the provider in assessing the smoker's motivation to quit smoking as well as guide an intervention (Prochaska, Redding, & Evers, 1997). The precontemplation phase is characterized by a lack of interest in smoking cessation in the foreseeable future and/or the next 6 months. An effective strategy is to understand the reasons for smoking as well as the fears about quitting. Inserting doubt about the benefits of smoking and increasing awareness of the risks associated with smoking without lecturing is appropriate. The contemplation stage is characterized by considering quitting smoking in the next

2–6 months. The intervention is focused on enhancing the motivation to quit. These individuals are considering quitting, and as providers we can facilitate tipping the balance toward smoking cessation by bringing out the reasons to change and enhancing self-efficacy. The preparation phase is characterized by getting ready to quit in the next 30 days. Often these individuals have made a quit attempt in the past year and are changing their smoking pattern. The intervention is aimed at enabling the tobacco user make a sustained quit attempt. The action phase is characterized by smoking abstinence in the last 6 months. Interventions are aimed at identifying barriers to maintaining the quit and enabling the individual to develop effective coping strategies. The last stage of change is maintenance, in which the individual has quit for more than 6 months. These individuals need to be aware of difficult situations in which a slip could occur (Abrams *et al.*, 2003).

An oncology nurse uses the 5 As—asking about smoking, advising the patient to stop smoking, assessing the willingness to make a quit attempt, assisting in the quit attempt, and referring the individual for follow-up, preferably to a tobacco treatment specialist (Clinical Practice Guidelines, 2000). A specialist focuses on both behavioral and pharmacologic approaches for smoking cessation. Utilizing a state tobacco quit line adds another layer of telephone support. The Agency for Health Care Policy and Research (AHCPR) has proposed a behavioral approach that includes the five Rs—relevance, risks, rewards, roadblocks, and repetition—and may be employed for those unwilling to quit.

In addition to the five As, other behavioral approaches include: setting a quit date; telling family, friends, and coworkers about quitting; anticipating challenges in quitting; and removing tobacco products from the home (Clinical Practice Guidelines, 2000).

The following pharmacotherapies have proved efficacious in helping the smoker quit and are considered first-line therapy: nicotine replacement therapy in the form of a patch, lozenge, gum, inhaler, or nasal spray; bupropion SR; and varenicline. Second-line medications that may provide benefit are clonidine and nortriptyline (Clinical Practice Guidelines, 2000).

It is imperative to support legislative actions that will help reduce the availability of tobacco products. This can be enabled by raising federal excise taxes on tobacco products and supporting the US Food and Drug Administration (FDA) in an effort to regulate tobacco products. Supporting smoke-free workplaces helps protect the public and increases awareness about the risks of secondhand smoke. In 1988 the Master Settlement between 46 state attorney generals and the tobacco industry resulted in funding to compensate past, present, and future costs associated with smoking. There is movement to regulate tobacco on the global level. The WHO Framework Convention on Tobacco Control (FCTC) was enacted in February 2005. This treaty is a coordinated global effort aimed at reducing tobacco use in hopes of reducing the world's leading preventable cause of death. Although 160 countries have ratified the treaty, the United States at the time of publication has not yet ratified the treaty (ASCO, 2009).

Smoking is associated with at least 15 types of cancer and is responsible for 30% of all cancer deaths. Smoking negatively influences the effectiveness of treatment, affects a patient's tolerance for treatment, increases the risk for a secondary cancer, and increases the risk for complications. As oncology nurses, it is crucial to assess for tobacco use at every visit, assist individuals to find help in quitting, and support legislative action to regulate the use of tobacco products.

References

Abrams, D. B., Niaura, R., Brown, R. A., Emmons, K. M., Goldstien, M. G., & Monti, P. M. (2003). In D. H. Barlow (Ed.), *The tobacco dependence treatment handbook*. New York: The Guilford Press.

American Society of Clinical Oncology. (2009). Tobacco cessation and quality cancer care. *Journal of Oncology Practice, 5*(1), 2–5.

Benowitz, N. L. (1996). Pharmacology of nicotine: addiction and therapeutics. *Annual Review Pharmacology and Toxicology, 36,* 597–613.

Federal Trade Commission. (2000). "Tar," nicotine, and carbon monoxide of the smoke of 1294 varieties of domestic cigarettes for the year 1998. Washington, DC: Federal Trade Commission.

Gritz, E. (2006). Smoking and smoking cessation in cancer patients. *Addiction, 86*(5), 549–554.

Hughes, J. R., & Hatsukami, D. (1992). The nicotine withdraw syndrome. A brief review and update. *International Journal of Smoking Cessation, 1,* 22–26.

National Institute of Drug Abuse Tobacco Addiction. Retrieved January 25, 2009, from http://www.nida.nih.gov/ResearchReports/Nicotine/Nicotine.html

Piasecki, T., Fiore, M., & Baker, T. (1997). Profiles in discouragement: Two studies of variability in the time course of smoking withdraw symptoms. *Journal of Abnormal Psychology, 107,* 238–251.

Prochaska, J. O., Redding, C. A., & Evers, K. E. (1997). The transtheoretical model and stages of change. In I. K. Glanz, F. M. Lewis, & B. K. Rimer (Eds.), *Health behaviors and health education*, 2nd ed. San Francisco: Jossey-Bass, 60–84.

Velicer, W. F., Fava, J. L., Prochaska, J. O., Abrams, D. B., Emmons, M., & Pierce, J. P. (1995). Distribution of smokers by stage in three representative samples. *Preventive Medicine, 24,* 401–411.

World Health Organization. (2008). Retrieved June 19, 2009, from http://www.who.int/features/factfiles/tobacco_epidemic/en/index.html

Bibliography

The Tobacco Use and Dependence Clinical Practice Guideline Panel, Staff and Consortiums Representatives, Treating Tobacco Use and Dependence: A U.S. Public Health Service Report. (2000). *Journal of the American Medical Association*. Retrieved January 31, 2009, from http://www.surgeongeneral.gov/tobacco/tobaqrg.htm

❦ COMPLEMENTARY THERAPIES

Paula A. Caron

Cancer survivors utilize complementary and alternative medicine (CAM) for a multitude of reasons. Some survivors are seeking a cure for advanced cancer, trying to maintain some modicum of control over their disease trajectory, or trying to maintain or restore health. Nurses often do much of the teaching with patients regarding procedures, medications, self-care, and maintenance of health. Therefore, they are often in the position of being asked about various complementary modalities and having to assess CAM use by their patients. In 2000, the Oncology Nursing Society published a position paper on CAM that has since been revised (Oncology Nursing Society, 2006). Among other things, this paper suggests that oncology nurses should increase their knowledge about CAM in regard to cancer care, assess patients' use of CAM, and document this use accordingly in the medical record (Oncology Nursing Society, 2006).

In 1993, Eisenberg *et al.* published an article in *The New England Journal of Medicine* that shocked the US medical community and changed the way it viewed complementary medicine modalities (Eisenberg *et al.*, 1993). Based on their survey data, the authors estimated that Americans had made more visits to complementary medicine care providers than to primary care physicians in 1990. Americans also paid more out-of-pocket money for complementary medicine visits than for hospital care in that same year. It was not that these modalities were new in and of themselves, but rather that a door had been opened into another realm of modalities to maintain health and treat illness. This trend has not changed; if anything, it has intensified. In 2007, the National Health Interview Survey (NHIS) reported that approximately 38% of adults (about 4 in 10) and 12% of children (about 1 in 9) are using some form of complementary or alternative medicine (Barnes, Bloom, & Nihan, 2007).

The National Center for Complementary and Alternative Medicine (NCCAM), defines CAM as "a group of diverse medical and health care systems, practices, and products that are not generally considered to be part of conventional medicine." They go on to describe three categories of CAM:

- *Complementary medicine* or therapy is in conjunction with conventional medicine
- *Alternative medicine* is used instead of conventional medicine
- *Integrative medicine* combines mainstream medical therapies and CAM

NCCAM recognizes four domains and one whole medical system:

- *Whole medical systems* are built on complete systems of theory or practice. Included are naturopathy, traditional Chinese medicine, Ayurveda, and homoeopathy.
- *Mind-body interventions* utilize the connection between the mind and body to effect a change on the body via influence from the mind. Such modalities as meditation, prayer, and therapies such as art, music, or dance are included.
- *Biologically based therapies* utilize substances found naturally including herbs, foods, and vitamins.
- *Manipulative and body-based practices* involve manipulation of parts of the body. They include therapeutic massage, chiropracty, and osteopathy.
- *Energy therapies* are comprised of two categories: Biofield therapies including therapeutic touch, Reiki, and qi gong. Bioelectromagnetic therapies using magnets or electricity

(National Center for Complementary and Alternative Medicine, 2009).

This section gives a broad overview of the more common modalities a nurse might be asked to provide information about to patients, including massage, acupuncture, Reiki, homeopathy, chiropracty, herbalism, therapeutic touch, naturopathy, Chinese medicine (also known as TCM), meditation, yoga, Qi gong, and tai chi. Although evidence is beginning to appear in the literature, many of these modalities have not been studied extensively. Through NCCAM, the federal government provides funds to rigorously research CAM modalities, train researchers, and educate the public and healthcare professionals about CAM.

Credentialing of providers remains a challenge, as there are no standards of care for many of the CAM modalities. Thus, it becomes the purview of individual institutions to decide who has been adequately trained to provide care to its patients. In the general community, there are no credentialing procedures; rather, word of mouth serves to identify the most skilled and effective of practitioners. Some states do have licensing requirements for practitioners of massage, acupuncture, naturopathy, and chiropracty. More often, the standards are set by the national organizational body of a particular discipline, which may require a practitioner to pass a standardized written and/or performance examination. There is no central agency to monitor or regulate practitioners of CAM; therefore, the nurse is referred to individual state government offices for licensing requirements or the national organization of a particular modality.

Acupuncture

Acupuncture involves the insertion of needles at points along the 12 meridians of energy that run along longitudinal lines in the body. These points correspond with various parts of the body, often organs.

Stimulation of these points allows chi, or life energy, to flow more freely and restore balance. There are different types of acupuncture, influenced by the country or origin of the practice, often China, Japan, or Korea.

Some practitioners incorporate other techniques with the acupuncture intended to enhance its effects. *Moxabustion* involves the burning of moxa, an herb that burns at very hot temperatures and is believed to further influence the acupuncture point. Electrical stimulation or *electroacupuncture,* of the needles with gentle electric current is also believed to enhance the effect of the acupuncture needles.

Acupressure, or a variant, *shiatsu massage,* are similar to acupuncture in that points along the meridians are stimulated but, unlike acupuncture, needles are not used. Rather, the points are stimulated with the fingers or hands.

Acupuncturists are trained in one of two ways, either by apprenticing with a master or through an academic master's program. Licensing legislation in some states is making the master's degree a requirement for entry.

Chiropracty

Chiropractic medicine is grounded in the belief that the human body has the capacity to heal itself and seeks balance. Through manual manipulation or adjustment of the bones and joints, often the spine, body parts are brought back into proper alignment to promote the flow of energy and resultant healing. Structure and function are closely related; thus, when the body is aligned structurally, the nervous system is allowed to function with efficiency, which promotes health.

Homeopathy

Homeopathy is based on the premise that "like cures like." Disease is a manifestation of an imbalance in the body as it naturally attempts to heal itself. Substances or remedies that produce disease symptoms in a well person can potentially cure the disease with similar symptoms in an ill person. Homeopathic remedies come from natural sources (plants, animals, and minerals) and are diluted into infinitesimal doses that are administered to the ill person after having been "proved" or tested in well volunteers. Energetically, homeopathic remedies stimulate the body's own abilities to heal it. The remedies are in such small dilutions that they are often without side effects (Lee, 2004; Rosser, 2004).

Massage

Massage may be the oldest form of medical care recorded. It involves manual stimulation of the body by stroking, rubbing, or kneading the tissues. There are many types of massage, but all are intended to manipulate muscle and connective tissue to enhance function, and promote relaxation and a sense of well-being (Gecsedi, 2002). Massage has not been proved to spread cancer cells as is sometimes thought. However, caution must be exercised in patients with thrombocytopenia, hypercoagulable states, or those who are at risk for fractures.

Meditation

Meditation has traditionally been grounded in spiritual tradition with the intention of spiritual growth or transcendence, but can also be used as a tool to achieve relaxation and mental clarity. It involves focusing of thought with intention to suspend the normally active human mind. In so doing, a state of deep relaxation is achievable. Benefits are also possible regarding control of perception of physical symptoms. With regular practice, an individual has the potential to change how he or she relates to the world and even the flow of thoughts that normally course through the mind.

Meditation can be done in a group setting, but whether as an individual or in a group, the focus is inward. Although traditionally done sitting or lying, meditation can be done while walking with a mindful focus on one thing at a time, such as counting steps or breaths.

Naturopathy

Naturopathy, an alternative medical system, attempts to support the body in its innate ability to heal itself. Natural healing approaches are utilized such as nutrition, vitamins and dietary supplements, herbs, homeopathy, and lifestyle counseling. Naturopathic physicians train in naturopathic medical schools with many of the core courses being the same as their allopathic medicine counterparts.

Qi Gong

Qi gong has its roots in Chinese medicine philosophy and uses physical movement, mental focus, and deep breathing with intention to promote healing and balance. The term qi gong loosely translates as "breath work," and is intended to move and manipulate qi (or chi or ki) in the body. The exercises are usually done in groups of repetitions.

Reiki

Reiki, an energy medicine practice, originated in Japan. The practitioner's hands are placed on or very near to various points on the receiver's body. It is believed that the practitioner serves as a conduit for energy from a higher source, which is transmitted to the receiver and in turn promotes relaxation and/or healing.

Reiki was rediscovered by Usui, a Japanese Buddhist monk in the 19th century, during his study of ancient healing texts. It came to the United States in the 1930s and began to be more widely used in the 1970s.

A Reiki practitioner is trained by being attuned by a Reiki master. There are three levels of attunement, each of which builds on the previous attunement, which is thought to open channels of higher vibration that allow Reiki or universal energy to flow to the recipient. The Reiki energy is thought to go where it is most needed in the body; the practitioner does not have to focus on a particular area. A Reiki treatment can occur over a few minutes or an hour. Because no particular equipment is needed, Reiki can be done on anyone, anywhere. There are no known side effects and it is safe for anyone.

Tai Chi

Tai chi originated in the Chinese martial arts. It involves moving the body in a routine with slow gentle movements. Focus is on the breath; thus, it is sometimes called moving meditation. While relaxing, Tai chi is also thought to promote health and well-being. It can be done in groups or individually.

Therapeutic Touch

Therapeutic Touch (TT) was developed by Dolores Krieger and Dora Kunz in the 1970s. According to Krieger, it is "the conscious intentional act of directing universal energy with the intent to help and heal" (Krieger, 1979; Potter, 2003). The TT practitioner's hands are passed over the patient while attempting to locate energy imbalances. The energy is then rebalanced by directing universal energy to the areas of imbalance with the intention of promoting healing and rebalancing.

Yoga

Yoga originated in India and is actually one of the six orthodox schools of Hindu philosophy. Breathing and physical postures are used to reach a meditative state, which results in promoting balance. Yoga can be performed as a solo practice or in a class. Many of the postures can be adapted to accommodate physical limitations.

❧ Summary

Cost may be an issue for some cancer survivors who wish to add CAM to their self-care because many insurers do not cover CAM modalities. Some insurance companies reimburse for chiropractic or naturopathic care, others reimburse for acupuncture. If the CAM practitioner is also an allopathic provider who has billing privileges, the services may be covered. Lastly, not to be underestimated is the benefit of many of these modalities to nurses who care for people with serious illnesses. The promotion of relaxation is crucial to prevent caregiver fatigue and burnout.

References

Barnes, B. M., Bloom, B., & Nihan, R. L. (2007). Complementary and Alternative Medicine Use Among Adults and Children: United States, 2007. National Health Statistics Report December 10, 2008, no 12, 1–24. Retrieved January 31, 2009, from http://nccam.nih.gov/news/2008/nhsr12.pdf

Eisenberg, D. M., Kessler, R. C., Foster, C., Norlock, F. E., Calkins, D. R., & Delbanco, T. L. (1993). Unconventional medicine in the United States. Prevalence, costs, and patterns of use. *New England Journal of Medicine, 328*(4), 246–252.

Gecsedi, R. A. (2002). Massage therapy for patients with cancer. *Clinical Journal of Oncology Nursing, 6*(1), 52–54.

Krieger, D. (1979). *The therapeutic touch: How to use your hands to help or to heal.* Englewood Cliffs, NJ: Prentice-Hall.

Lee, C. O. (2004). Homeopathy in cancer care: Part II—Continuing the practice of "like curing like." *Clinical Journal of Oncology Nursing, 8*(3), 327–330.

National Center for Complementary and Alternative Medicine (2009). *What is CAM?* Retrieved January 31, 2009, from http://nccam.nih.gov/health/whatiscam/overview.htm

Oncology Nursing Society. (2006). *The Use of Complementary, Alternative, and Integrative Therapies in Cancer Care* [Position statement]. Retrieved January 31, 2009, from http://www.ons.org/publications/positions/ComplementaryTherapies.shtml

Potter, P. (2003). What are the distinctions between reiki and therapeutic touch? *Clinical Journal of Oncology Nursing, 7*(1), 89–91.

Rosser, C. (2004). Homeopathy in cancer care: Part I—an introduction to "like curing like." *Clinical Journal of Oncology Nursing, 8*(3), 324–326.

Bibliography

Ferrell, B. R., & Coyle, N. (2006). *Textbook of palliative nursing.* New York: Oxford University Press.

Lee, C. O. (2004). Translational research in cancer complementary and alternative medicine: The National Cancer Institute's Best Case Series Program. *Clinical Journal of Oncology Nursing, 8*(2), 212–241.

Lee, C. O. (2004). Clinical Trials in Cancer Part I. Biomedical, complementary, and alternative medicine: finding active trials and results of closed trials. *Clinical Journal of Oncology Nursing, 8*(5), 531–535.

Lee, C. O. (2004). Clinical Trials in Cancer Part II. Biomedical, complementary, and alternative medicine: Significant issues. *Clinical Journal of Oncology Nursing, 8*(6), 670–674.

Hospice and Palliative Nurses Association. (2008). Position statement: Complementary Therapies in Palliative Care Nursing Practice. Retrieved January 31, 2009, from http://www.hpna.org/DisplayPage.aspx?Title=Position%20Statements

Decker, G. M., & Abdallah-Baran, R. (2003). Nurturing spirit through complementary cancer care. *Clinical Journal of Oncology Nursing, 7*(4), 468–470.

National Center for Complementary and Alternative Medicine. (2009). *What Is CAM?* Retrieved January 31, 2009, from http://nccam.nih.gov/health/whatiscam/overview.htm

Additional Resources

American Association of Naturopathic Physicians (AANP)
601 Valley Street, Suite 105

Seattle, WA 98109
Phone: (206) 328-8510
http://www.naturopathic.org

American Holistic Nurses Association
323 N. San Francisco St.
Suite 201
Flagstaff, AZ 86001
(800) 278-2462
http://www.ahna.org

Consumerlab.com
Independent testing of health and nutritional products
http://www.consumerlab.com

International Chiropractors Association
1110 N Glebe Rd
Suite 650
Arlington, VA 22201
Phone: (703) 528-5000; Toll free (800) 423-4690
fax: 703-528-5023
http://www.chiropractic.org/

National Cancer Institute (NCI)
http://www.cancer.gov

NCI Office of Cancer Complementary and Alternative Medicine
http://www3.cancer.gov/occam

National Center for Complementary and Alternative Medicine
http://www.nccam.nih.gov

National Center for Homeopathy
801 North Fairfax Street, Suite 306
Alexandria, VA 22314
Phone: (703) 548-7790
http://www.homeopathic.org

National Certification Board for Therapeutic Massage and Bodywork
8201 Greensboro Drive, Suite 300
McLean, VA 22102
Phone: (800) 296-0664
http://www.ncbtmb.com

National Certification Commission for Acupuncture and Oriental Medicine (NCCA)
1424 16th Street NW
Suite 501
Washington, DC 20036

Nurse Healers—Professional Associates International
Box 419
Craryville, NY 12521
Phone: (518) 325-1185; Toll Free (877) 32NHPAI
Fax: (509) 693-3537
http://www.therapeutic-touch.org

Office of Dietary Supplements (ODS), NIH
http://www.ods.od.nih.gov

❦ BONE HEALTH

Laura Urquhart

❦ Introduction

One of the most prevalent but invisible long-term side effects of cancer treatment is bone loss. Cancer treatment-induced bone loss (CTIBL) can be specifically associated with some types of anticancer therapy. Cancer survivors may not understand and realize how their treatment places them at increased risk of fracture, which can significantly impact their quality of life and threaten their survival. This complication is most frequently seen in breast and prostate cancer survivors. However, any cancer survivor should have bone health evaluated as part of his or her follow-up care.

Bone loss has been categorized into two conditions: osteopenia and osteoporosis. Osteopenia is the loss of bone mass, whereas osteoporosis is a condition in which the bones are thinned and weakened. Both are treatable conditions that may occur as a result of cancer care and/or are caused by risk factors unrelated to cancer care, such as menopause and genetic conditions. Bones undergo a continual process of repair called remodeling. Bone remodeling is characterized by resorption of old bone osteoclasts and formation of new bone by osteoblasts. This process continues throughout life to maintain structure and mineral integrity. During the normal aging process, the reduction of gonadal hormones, such as during menopause, causes bone loss to occur more rapidly than bone formation in older men and women. This results in a decrease in bone mineral density (BMD), increased bone loss, and a resulting increased risk of fracture. The World Health Organization (WHO) has established guidelines for interpreting the results of tests to measure bone density such as DEXA scans that measure BMD (Table 6-3).

TABLE 6-3   WHO Diagnostic Criteria = T Score

Normal = ≥1.0
Osteopenia (decreased bone mass) = between −1.0 and −2.5
Osteoporosis = ≥2.5

These criteria apply *only* to white postmenopausal women.

Some cancer therapies induce hypogonadism (e.g., androgen deprivation for prostate cancer and aromatase inhibitors for hormone receptor-positive breast cancers and hormonal agents), other treatment protocols include the use of corticosteroids and/or thyroid-stimulating hormone suppressive therapy, both of which influence bone health. Patients receiving cancer treatments may also experience alterations in diet resulting in altered absorption of vital nutrients, such as calcium and vitamin D.

Cancer survivors who are at risk for bone loss should have BMD testing done at scheduled intervals. Some healthcare providers will perform additional testing to assess kidney and liver function. During the evaluation, serum chemistries may also be used to measure levels of substances that play a role in bone health such as parathyroid hormone, thyroid stimulating hormone (TSH), vitamin D, serum calcium, phosphorus, and alkaline phosphates level. (Pfeilschifter & Deil, 2000).

Oncology nurses can assist in identifying those survivors at risk for CTIBL by identifying preexisting risk factors (Table 6-4). They can also provide education regarding the results of BMD, and the importance of weight-bearing exercise, as well as the importance of adherence to adequate intake of calcium and vitamin D. Resistance and weight

TABLE 6-4   Lifestyle Risk Factors

Anorexia

Diet low in calcium and vitamin D

Sedentary lifestyle

Lack of weight-bearing exercises

Cigarette smoking

Alcohol consumption

Use of steroids and anticonvulsants

bearing exercises and a daily intake of 1200–1500 mg of calcium and 600–800 IU of vitamin D should be recommended (Hillner *et al.*, 2003) (Tables 6-5 and 6-6).

Now that there are more than 12 million cancer survivors, and an aging population, evaluation and management of CTIBL will continue to be a significant healthcare issue. Oncology nurses can assist in identifying

TABLE 6-5   Primary Risk Factors

Female gender

Older age

Estrogen deficiency

White or Asian race

Low body weight and mass

Family history of osteoporosis

History of fracture in adulthood

TABLE 6-6   Bisphosphonates

Medication	Brand name	Dosage	Side effects
Alendronate	Fosamax	10 mg PO daily or 70 mg PO weekly	Gastrointestinal irritation, myalgias, and arthralgias
Ibandronate	Boniva	150 mg PO once a month 2.5 mg PO daily	Gastrointestinal irritation, myalgia, arthralgias
Risedronate	Actonel	5 mg PO daily or 35 mg PO weekly	Same as with Fosamax
Calcitonin nasal spray	Miacalcin	200 units intranasally daily	Rhinitis and epistaxis
Zoledronic acid	Reclast	4 mg IV q 6 mos	Flulike symptoms, nausea and vomiting, fever, flushing, and decreased appetite. Must check creatinine. Prolonged use ONJ
Teriparatide	Forteo	20–25 mcg SC	Tenderness at injection site Muscle leg cramps

those survivors with risk factors and provide ongoing education on lifestyle changes to promote bone health through exercise and diet. Oncology nurses may also assess for medication adherence and medication toxicity. Lastly, they can reinforce treatment recommendations to counteract CTIBL, thereby impacting the overall quality of life for survivors.

References

Hillner, B. E., Ingle, J. N., Chlebowski, R.T., Gralow, J.,Yee, G. C., Janjan N. A., *et al*. (2003). American Society of clinical Oncology 2003 update on the role of bisphosphonates in bone health in women with breast cancer. *Journal of Clinical Oncology, 21,* 4042–4057.

Pfeilschifter, J., & Diel, I. J. (2000). Osteoposis due to cancer treatment. Pathogenesis and management. *Journal of Clinical Oncology, 18,* 1570–1593.

Bibliography

American Society of Clinical Oncology: ASCO.org

Brufsky, A., Harker, J. T., Beck, R., Carroll, E., Tan-Chiu, C., Seidler, L. *et al*. (2005). Zoledronic acid effectively inhibits cancer treatment-induced bone loss (CTIBL) in postmenopausal women (PMW) with early breast cancer (Bca) receiving adjuvant letrozole (let): 12 mos. BMD results of the Z-fast trial. *Journal of Clinical Oncology, 23*(16), 533.

Gnant, M., Hausmaninger, H., Samonigg, H., Mlineritsch, B.,Taucher, S., Luschin-Ebengreuth, G., *et al*. (2002). Changes in bone mineral density caused by anastrozole or tamoxifen in combination with goserelin as adjuvant treatment for hormone receptor-positive breast cancer. Results of a randomized trial [Abstract]. *Breast Cancer Research and Treatment, 76*(1), S31.

Kuehn, B. M. (2005). Better osteoporosis management a priority: Impact predicted to soar with aging population. *JAMA, 293,* 2453–2458.

Maxwell, C., & Viale, P. H. (2005). Cancer treatment–induced bone loss in patients with breast or prostate cancer. *Oncology Nursing Forum, 32,* 589–601.

National Osteoporosis Foundation: http://nof.org

Swenson, K. K., Henly, S. J., Shapiro, A. C., & Schroeder, L. M. (2005). Interventions to prevent loss of bone mineral density in women receiving chemotherapy for breast cancer. *Clinical Journal of Oncology Nursing, 9*(2), 177–184.

CHAPTER SEVEN

Communication and Interpersonal Relationships

Lisa Kennedy Sheldon

Introduction

Being a person with a cancer diagnosis changes relationships at home, in the workplace, and in the community. One of the biggest challenges for many cancer survivors is not treatment itself, but communicating with others about their disease. In any setting, people with whom they have relationships may react differently; be quieter than usual, watch them more closely, check in more frequently, create more distance, or even act as if nothing has happened. Sometimes survivors have the added burden of making others feel more at ease about their diagnosis. At other times, they have to learn to accept assistance from others as one way to make other people feel more helpful. Survivors have to learn a new way of communicating with others after a diagnosis of cancer.

Communication is especially important after a cancer diagnosis. Talking about the diagnosis, treatment, and life during survivorship is an important part of creating the "new normal" for a cancer survivor. Without communication, survivors may feel lonely and isolated, with some becoming anxious or clinically depressed. Oncology nurses are ideally positioned to help patients and survivors move along the cancer journey, assess their adaptation, and help them approach survivorship with the necessary resources. Nurses often spend extended periods of time with people during treatments, hospitalizations, or follow-up care. Concerns regarding family relationships, jobs, and even roles in the community may arise spontaneously during visits. Addressing these issues facilitates adaptation and performance in these roles and develops a solid foundation for care during survivorship.

Spouses and Partners

Cancer survivors notice how their diagnosis affects their relationships. Spouses and partners of survivors, whether in a marriage or long-term relationship, often feel the impact of the diagnosis intensely. Because these relationships are a source of emotional support for both partners, a change in one partner affects the other. Both partners may face feelings of fear, anxiety, and anger, but they can often strengthen their relationship during this shared challenge. They both will experience changes in many aspects of their relationship, including roles and responsibilities, physical and emotional needs, and changes in sexuality and intimacy. In any partnership, each partner takes on certain roles and responsibilities, such as finances, social planning, childcare, and income generation. Although it is often accepted that cancer treatment will change the patient's functioning, it is probably less well understood that some changes might be present for the long term, requiring more permanent changes in roles. Some problems, such as fatigue, may extend into survivorship, making it difficult to work full time or requiring a shift in responsibilities such as housework.

Survivors and their partners may have to approach some difficult conversations. It may require a new set of communication skills to discuss these challenging issues. Examples of these conversations cited on the LIVESTRONG Web site are:

- Living with uncertainty
- Stress
- Feelings of guilt
- Financial difficulties
- Dealing with fear of recurrence
- Changes in outlook on life and death
- Recognizing symptoms of recurrence or other physical problems
- Losses of all kinds: job, friends, abilities
- Changing roles and responsibilities
- New compromises that need to be made
- Feeling overwhelmed
- Anger

Because some of these conversations are heavy with emotions such as fear and sadness, couples may find their old communication patterns strained and ineffective. Oncology nurses, by recognizing that these challenges exist, can ask survivors and their partners about concerns within their relationship. The first time they bring up this topic, survivors may not acknowledge the issues because of their focus on treatment and physical concerns. However, by opening the door, the partners may bring their concerns to the nurse at another visit. The nurse can further assess the issues in the relationship, normalize some experiences, and refer couples for further counseling as needed.

The physical and emotional needs of the survivor may change during and after active treatment. Some survivors need ongoing help to meet their physical needs, such as help with bathing, requiring the partner to assume new caregiving roles. Some people have more emotional needs and require ongoing emotional support and reassurance, especially during times of increasing vulnerability such as follow-up testing or new symptoms. The need for sexual intimacy may change because of the side effects of treatment, decreased libido, and/or ongoing symptoms such as fatigue. Open communication between partners facilitates adjustment and may build on the strengths of the relationship as both partners assume new roles.

Couples often have to adjust to a new sense of future after a cancer diagnosis. The prospect of a potentially life-shortening diagnosis is very difficult for many couples, requiring readjustment of future plans and a resorting of priorities. When the time of crisis around diagnosis is over and the treatment is finished, previous issues in the partnership may resurface. Couples often benefit from talking with a social worker, therapist, and/or pastoral counselor to re-evaluate priorities and establish short- and long-term goals. As couples work together they often feel more connected; strengthening their relationship and improving the quality of their time together.

Family Life

A cancer diagnosis affects more than the survivor; it also affects the family members. Siblings, parents, and more distant relations all feel the impact of the diagnosis. Often the patient/survivor has to take the lead in beginning the conversation, because family members may feel at a loss for words or not know where to begin for fear of upsetting the survivor. For some family members, the diagnosis of cancer is a frightening reality, one in which the same thing could happen to them. Or perhaps it brings up memories of others in their lives who have had cancer or loved ones they have lost. Often, cancer survivors have the surprising job of making family members feel more comfortable with the diagnosis and opening up conversations about their health.

Of special note is the effect of a parent's cancer diagnosis on his or her children. Children fear losing their parents, a frightening prospect even for adult children. Even very young children notice changes and hear whispers or silenced conversations. Honest information in simple messages helps them to understand changes in appearance, such as hair loss, or decreased energy. The survivor may not to be able to continue in all the activities of parenting he or she previously engaged in, but continues to be important in the lives of his or her children.

Noticing changes in children's behavior may signal the need for more open conversations. Children may behave differently; young children may become clingier or adolescents may have a shorter temper. Survivors can spend more time with their children, encouraging them to talk about their concerns and feelings. Simple facts about treatment and side effects may make the unknown more understandable and allay some of their fears. Other times, honesty may be more appropriate when preparing for permanent changes in functioning or shortened futures. Parents are not alone when facing tough conversations with their children. In addition to healthcare providers, social workers, and pastoral counseling, programs such as CLIMB (Children's Lives Include Moments of Bravery) provide ongoing group sessions to help children explore their feelings about a parent with cancer and improve their mental health. Often, supportive services help both children and their parents adjust to the impact of a cancer diagnosis.

❈ Work Relationships

A cancer diagnosis is often accompanied by changing relationships, including those in the workplace. Although the time around active treatment may focus on side effects and temporary changes in functioning, re-entering social and professional life can be accompanied by many fears: worry about being out in the world with an increased risk of infection; not having enough energy to get through a work day; or anxiety about not being able to think clearly because of "chemobrain" or memory loss. There are often fears about changed attitudes from coworkers regarding competence, discrimination, or being treated differently. Survivors often worry about losing their jobs or healthcare insurance. These worries create uncertainty and fear that increases stress in the survivor. Open communication may be the best approach, allowing the survivor to talk about his or her health and address the concerns of coworkers and employers. Legal protection is offered for those with concerns about discrimination (See Chapter 9 on Coordination of Care).

Friends

Many cancer survivors feel distant from peers who have not had the same experience. They have had to review their priorities and values and often faced life-and-death questions in a way that their friends may not. Friends may vary in their responses to the cancer survivor. Some friends may always see the survivor as "sick," even if the cancer was treated long ago. At other times, support comes from surprising places, even from friends who have not previously been supportive. Friends may become closer as they help the cancer survivor by listening, supporting, helping with daily activities, or providing fun and entertainment. A diagnosis of cancer can bring out new dimensions in friendships that are sustaining for many cancer survivors.

Support in Survivorship

Living with uncertainty is often part of reality for cancer survivors. By talking with others, whether friends, family, or in support groups, survivors can discuss their concerns and fears, and set realistic goals for the future. Often they have a sense of accomplishment from facing the diagnosis of cancer. ASCO's patient Web site, People Living With Cancer, reviews some common responses to finishing treatment and sources of support. When people finish treatment, they do not see their healthcare providers as often. Healthcare providers, especially nurses, are often a source of support for patients. They normalize some of the patient's responses and symptoms and provide further assessment and referral for treatment as needed. When survivors face their symptoms and concerns at home, they often feel removed and debate calling their healthcare providers, unsure of the importance of their issues. They may experience sadness and loss for what "might have been" if they had not had this diagnosis, or perhaps feel their body "failed" them.

Many survivors express a desire to help other people with cancer. Support groups have been created by survivors, social workers, and nurses to help others adapt to their changed reality after diagnosis. By sharing their experiences with others who have been down a similar path, survivors not only help themselves, but also help others.

Bibliography

CLIMB (Children's Lives Include Moments of Bravery). (2009). Children's Treehouse Foundation. Retrieved January 26, 2009, from http://www.childrenstreehousefdn.org/ourroll3.html

LIVESTRONG. (2009). Lance Armstrong Foundation: Communicating with your partner. Retrieved on January 26, 2009, from http://www.livestrong.org/site/c.khLXK1PxHmF/b.2660643/k.4BD3/Communicating_With_Your_Partner.htm

People Living With Cancer. (2009). American Society of Clinical Oncology's patient Web site. Retrieved on January 28, 2009, from www.PLWC.org

Relationships and Family Life. (2009). Cancer.net. Retrieved January 26, 2009, from http://www.cancer.net/patient/Coping/Relationships+and+Cancer/Family+Life

Sheldon, L. K. (2008). *Communication for nurses: Talking with patients,* (2nd ed.). Sudbury, MA: Jones and Bartlett Publishers.

CHAPTER EIGHT

Spiritual Growth and Survivorship

Karen A. Skalla and Claire Pace

🔖 Introduction

A diagnosis of cancer may affect the core personhood of an individual in a variety of ways. Some individuals may integrate it as a part of life, and therefore resume normal behavior patterns and activities (Vachon, 2008). Many identify the diagnosis as a crisis. This crisis can provide an opportunity for spiritual transformation and growth. Cancer survivors may undergo a process of redefining their personal sense of self. During this pivotal experience, they may find themselves forced to re-order goals and priorities because of physical disability or role changes. Alternatively, they may choose this reordering and find themselves motivated in new ways or toward new opportunities (Vachon, 2008). Still others may struggle to derive a sense of meaning or purpose in their illness experience, requiring them to redefine or reframe their faith in a higher power.

The process toward spiritual growth can be both powerful and painful. A person's entire identity may come into question and be redesigned. Strong patient–provider relationships developed during the course of cancer treatment offer providers of cancer care a unique opportunity to establish a connection with which to assess and assist survivors' spiritual development and growth. Additionally, personal insight gained through this growth can facilitate spiritual resilience and strength with which a cancer *patient* can face his or her disease as a cancer *survivor*. It is the responsibility of those who care for these survivors to support their cancer experience and find ways to assist in the transformation process.

Spirituality and Spiritual Distress

What exactly is meant by the term *spirituality*? Many definitions exist. The authors propose a working definition for spirituality as a sense of peace, purpose, love, and connection to others, a concept of ultimate meaning and purpose to life that provides the organizing center of our lives from which our hopes, fears, and questions arise. The way in which we as individuals define spirituality develops as our awareness of our own spirituality deepens. Human beings have a fundamental need to seek meaning and fulfillment in order to provide purpose and coherence in an individual's life (Frankl, 1945).

Spiritual distress or spiritual suffering can be described as an emotional state in which a person is unable to fulfill basic human needs for love, hope, purpose, and connection with others, or a situation in which there is conflict between an individual's core beliefs and personal experience (Bartel, 2004). Spiritual distress is not uncommon in patients with serious illness (Albaugh, 2003; Cornette, 2005). It is an unrecognized phenomenon (Sulmasy, 2006) despite the fact that this group is likely to experience spiritual distress and is unlikely to have their spiritual needs assessed (Hermann, 2006; Kub *et al.*, 2003). Spirituality is an integral component of the quality of life (QOL) model, which encompasses physical, social, psychological, and spiritual domains with respect to survivorship (B. R. Ferrell, Dow, Leigh, Ly, & Gulasekaram, 1995). Spirituality can positively affect QOL (Leak, Hu, & King, 2008; McGrath, 2004). As predicted by Ferrell *et al.*'s model (B. R. Ferrell *et al.*, 2005; B. R. Ferrell *et al.*, 1995), high levels of spiritual distress may negatively affect QOL.

As people with cancer face potentially life-threatening illness, they must negotiate some of the most spiritually-threatening questions central to human existence. Survivors can respond either positively (spiritual growth) or negatively (spiritual distress) to this threat. The body of literature describing how people respond is beginning to grow. The positive impact of life-threatening illness has been explored by McGrath (2004). Individuals who experienced life-threatening illness had increased confidence and assertiveness manifested as being less dependent on others and finding it easier to assert personal needs, along with an increased awareness of physical needs. Interpersonal outcomes determined that patients were less judgmental and more compassionate, had a desire to live life to the fullest, changed work values, and developed a stronger connection with family and friends. Lastly, they had a sense of increased respect from others. These outcomes demonstrate considerable spiritual growth, which can build solid core resiliency.

Spiritual care cannot be directed simply to the individual diagnosed with cancer. Caregivers of survivors have their own journey to undertake, and it may prove effective to target interventions toward those who care for people diagnosed with cancer. In a qualitative study (Ka'opua, Gotay, & Boehm, 2007) focused on spouses of men with prostate cancer, spiritually-based resources facilitated adaptation to the crisis of diagnosis in the four core areas of marriage and intimacy, personal growth, health-related attitudes and behaviors, and community connections. Spouses who adapted were able to develop an "embracing" spirit and commonly felt a connection with a sacred source. Spiritual-based resources were used to sustain hope in facing change, loss, and pressure for problem solving, as well as discerning spiritual lessons in adverse events. Spirituality functioned as a cultural force, enabling the spouses to view themselves in relation to changing life events—they were able to make meaning that translated into coping.

⊗ Spirituality and the Survivor's Search for Meaning

Making meaning from an experience of cancer can have a profound impact on spiritual growth in the cancer survivor. Meaning for the cancer survivor includes "one's sense of purpose in life, the belief in the value of life, the coherent explanation of life events, well-being, and spirituality" (Jim, Purnell, Richardson, Golden-Kreutz, & Andersen, 2006, p. 1360). Therefore, meaning in this context can be defined as having many components and is present when one has a sense of purpose, coherence, and fulfillment in a life that is perceived to have value (Jim *et al.*, 2006).

These components—spiritual beliefs, spiritual practices, and the construction of meanings—are grounded in a relationship with a source that is perceived as sacred, and (McGrath, 2004) can act synergistically to create meaning. It is the content and context of meaning that is important to QOL, not simply the idea of having meaning (Clarke, 2006). Functionally, coping and spirituality are both meaning-centered processes that involve a search for significance in life events. For cancer survivors, the search for significance begins at diagnosis and continues throughout the cancer experience. It may change over time as their perceptions shift with life experience.

Park and Folkman (1997) identify two specific types of meaning. *Global meaning* represents beliefs about the order of life or the universe, as well as personal life goals and purpose. *Situational Meaning*, in contrast, is the interaction of a person's global beliefs within the context of a particular life experience. When a person undergoes a stressful life experience such as cancer (Jim *et al.*, 2006), his or her ability to find congruence between the two types of meaning determines whether or not that survivor feels stressed. Therefore, meaning making is the response to the impulse for congruence. The ability of survivors to find situational meaning in the experience that is congruent with their global meaning has been associated with better adjustment and subsequently less spiritual distress.

Many spiritual practices are used in the process of making meaning. Patients have reported regular use of spirituality and religion to cope with their diagnosis and treatment (Jim *et al.*, 2006). Many cancer survivors can find spiritual comfort by perceiving the experience of illness in terms of a positive spiritual journey (McGrath, 2004; Rancour, 2008). This journey may include concepts such as: Everything happens for a reason, having a sense of being "chosen" for this experience, the need to see illness as a challenge and the need to take personal responsibility to overcome that challenge, and finally having a sense of personal growth and pride in meeting that challenge (McGrath, 2004).

❧ Spiritual Care of the Cancer Survivor

The spiritual dimension of care is the fundamental act of "being with" another in need. Spiritual assessment of the patient with cancer is a delicate task that must be done with sensitivity and acceptance. It does not require completion in one session but may evolve over time. The issue of time is critical for clinicians, and can be a major barrier toward completing a spiritual assessment. Clinicians are ideally positioned to provide an opportunity to discover such meaning through spiritual care, as they are directly involved in those experiences that profoundly impact the patient's life (Rumbold, 2003).

Spiritual distress may be overlooked in the clinical setting. Little has been written about how to screen patients to ascertain who needs a more in-depth assessment (Kub *et al.*, 2003). Cancer survivors have little time to raise the issue of spirituality within the context of clinic visits that, in the current healthcare environment, are becoming increasingly short. Currently, there is no definitive and adequate process by which spiritual assessment is undertaken with outpatients, and assessment in this setting is generally limited to the question of a patient's religious preference. Most commonly a patient is referred to the Chaplaincy office either when the individual directly expresses the need for help, or when distress in the patient is clearly recognized. Clinical staff, for a variety of reasons, rarely undertake a spiritual assessment or feel prepared to deliver spiritual care (McEwen, 2005) when faced with spiritual questions posed by their patients. Questions repeatedly important to patients are (Miller, 2005): Why is this happening to me? What is the meaning of my life? What happens when we die? When faced with such questions from a patient, most caregivers refer the patient to Chaplaincy for pastoral care. This is entirely appropriate because of the specialized knowledge and role of the clinically trained chaplain; however, such resources may not always be available at the moment when they are most needed, nor are they common in the outpatient setting. However, when Chaplaincy resources exist, the cooperative attention of the clinician and the chaplain can enhance the benefit of spiritual care to patients (McClung, Grossoehme, & Jacobson, 2006).

In a recent study (Miller, 2005), only 37% of patients received help in dealing with spiritual questions during their cancer experience—two thirds from their pastor, and one third from family members. Functional assessment scores were significantly higher in those patients who received help from either source, as compared with those who did not receive help. Eighty percent wanted their physician to ask about emotional problems, and fifty-nine percent wanted them to ask if they needed spiritual help. As oncology caregivers we are obligated, as part of our holistic care, to acknowledge and encourage exploration of spiritual issues if our patients choose to share that journey with us. Some providers may not be prepared to respond to this opportunity, or they may not agree with this responsibility, and in fact may see it as a burden (Walter, 2002). However, in such cases they should be able to assess and actively pursue resources for referral.

Assessment of the cancer survivor for spiritual concerns can be accomplished in a variety of ways. Although comprehensive assessment is the role of chaplaincy, a variety of tools are available to the healthcare provider that can assist in this process and provide guidance for intervention by healthcare providers. Although one standard does not yet exist, many models and tools from various disciplines have been developed and utilized in survivor populations. Screening assessment of the individual who has faced cancer should include both their strengths and their potential for growth within the personal domains of values, vocation, social support, creativity, and transcendence (Skalla & McCoy, 2006). Strengths that may become evident upon assessment are interpersonal growth and a deepened sense of spirituality, enhanced appreciation for life both in the sense of its fragility and uncertainty as well as its inherent value, reordered life priorities, increased empathy and compassion for others, increased self-esteem, and a greater sense of meaning in life.

Several tools have focused on specific information according to the interests of the discipline within which they were developed. An assessment developed specifically for use in cancer survivor populations by Ferrell, the Quality of Life Cancer Patient/Survivor Tool (QOL-CS) (Dow, Ferrell, & Leigh, 1996; B. Ferrell, Hassey-Dow, & Grant, 1995) depicts spirituality as an integral component of the QOL model, which encompasses physical, social, psychological, and spiritual domains with respect to survivorship. Ferrell has extrapolated that model to patients undergoing active treatment (B. R. Ferrell *et al.*, 2005). The Functional Assessment of Chronic Illness Therapy- Spiritual Well Being Scale (FACIT-Sp) (Peterman, Fitchett, Brady, Hernandez, & Cella, 2002), is a well-known and tested tool that was created specifically to assess for spirituality and has been used extensively in cancer populations.

Many psychological tools have been used to assist in describing the experience of patients with cancer. The sense of meaning in life can be explicitly assessed using the Meaning in Life Scale (MiLS) developed by Jim *et al.* (2006) to elicit a sense of the individual's spirituality in the context of harmony and peace, life purpose, and goals, as well as confusion and lessened meaning for those who are struggling. The Post Traumatic Growth Inventory (PTGI) (Tedeschi & Calhoun, 1996) has been tested extensively for reliability and validity and successfully applied to cancer survivors (Jaarsma, Pool, Sanderman, & Ranchor, 2006). Unlike many other tools, this assessment uses a positive approach to look for individual growth in the context of a traumatic experience such as cancer.

The Spiritual Symptom Scale as part of the BioPsychoSocio-Spiritual Inventory (BioPSSI) was used to look at spiritual symptoms and the important relationship to utilization of healthcare services (Katerndahl, 2008) and healthcare outcomes. Spiritual symptoms (alone or in interaction with physical symptoms) were particularly important to extreme use of healthcare services and life satisfaction. Among best-fit models, spiritual symptoms alone were significantly associated with any mental health use, fair–poor health status, and life lacking meaning. These findings demonstrate how spiritual symptoms can act synergistically with other symptom dimensions to affect physical and mental health.

It is critically important that spirituality be a part of the comprehensive assessment of cancer survivors. Maintaining a positive attitude may be the most difficult part of the cancer journey, but it can become a transformative experience that translates into profound spiritual growth. When successfully negotiated, the journey can expand a person's repertoire of thoughts and actions to be able to engage in new ways of thinking and behaving creatively and help people to see coherence in life events such as cancer in order to foster a belief in how full of meaning life is (Jim *et al.*, 2006). Meaninglessness may contribute to decreased motivation. Statements such as, "Life is hopeless" or "I can't do anything about this" reflect lack of meaning for the individual to structure his or her life into a new normal.

Rancour uses Transitions Theory (Bridges, 2004) to provide structure to survivors when talking about how to remake their life into a new normal (Rancour, 2008). The first stage, Endings, is characterized by letting go of old relationships (with healthcare providers) and roles (as an ill person), even if the transition is positive (cancer is cured). This implies a process of grief, sadness, and anger as this stage is left behind. Support for this mourning comes from "being with" rather than "fixing" on the part of the nurse. The survivor's effort to experience and tolerate his or her most difficult emotions allows that individual to heal and move on, rather than remain stuck in his or her own distress.

The second stage, Neutral Zone, is characterized by a sense of confusion, chaos, and anxiety. This stage is characterized by a lack of structure. Survivors are struggling to define a new normal. In that process, a loss of identity can trigger discomfort, anxiety, and panic. They need to be assured that their feelings are normal and that the new identity will emerge once it is formed. Encouraging survivors to attend to this distress by caring for themselves allows them to tolerate suffering within themselves and translates later into compassion for others. Cultivating silence and reflection on the emerging identity through journaling, meditating, or use of ritual may be helpful (Rancour, 2008).

Finally, a New Beginning stage is reached, in which survivors are ready to move on and take advantage of new opportunities. Nurses are encouraged to resist trying to "fix" in this stage, and instead assist in identifying new skills, asking about new life meaning, and encouraging survivors to try new things (Rancour, 2008).

❀ Summary

Fixing is the result of training in a biomedical model, and facing the limitations of medicine can lead to a loss of hope for us as providers who strive always to fix illness and suffering. Spiritual pain cannot be fixed in the way that physical pain can be fixed; however, the willingness and ability to provide spiritual care ameliorates the frustration we frequently experience when physical care alone can no longer alleviate suffering. The act of providing spiritual care helps nurses to reconnect with the reason they chose to work in oncology nursing. It addresses that part of them that chose to extend beyond the boundaries of themselves to give to others. It is not just a job; for many it is a vocation (Ramondetta & Sills, 2004). However, keeping this perspective under the increasing demands of the current healthcare environment is a formidable challenge (Puchalski & Romer, 2000). This challenge must be met in order for us to survive and thrive as healers in oncology nursing.

References

Albaugh, J. A. (2003). Spirituality and life-threatening illness: a phenomenologic study. *Oncology Nursing Forum Online, 30*(4), 593–598.

Bartel, M. (2004). What is spiritual? What is spiritual suffering? *The Journal of Pastoral Care & Counseling, 58*(3), 187–201.

Bridges, W. (2004). *Transitions: Making sense of life's changes.* New York: DaCapo Press.

Clarke, J. (2006). A discussion paper about "meaning" in the nursing literature on spirituality: An interpretation of meaning as "ultimate concern" using the work of Paul Tillich. *International Journal of Nursing Studies, 43,* 915–921.

Cornette, K. (2005). The imponderable: A search for meaning. For whenever I am weak, I am strong. *International Journal of Palliative Nursing, 11*(3), 147–153.

Dow, K., Ferrell, B., & Leigh, S. (1996). An evaluation of the quality of life among long-term survivors of breast cancer. *Breast Cancer Research, 39,* 261–273.

Ferrell, B., Hassey-Dow, K., & Grant, M. (1995). Measurement of the quality of life in Cancer Survivors. *Quality of Life Research, 4,* 523–531.

Ferrell, B. R., Cullinane, C. A., Ervin, K., Melancon, C., Uman, G. C., & Juarez, G. (2005). Perspectives on the impact of ovarian cancer: Women's views of Quality of Life. *Oncology Nursing Forum, 32*(6), 1143–1149.

Ferrell, B. R., Dow, K. H., Leigh, S., Ly, J., & Gulasekaram, P. (1995). Quality of life in long-term cancer survivors. *Oncology Nursing Forum, 22,* 915–922.

Frankl, V. (1945). *Man's search for meaning.* Boston: Beacon Press.

Hermann, C. (2006). Development and testing of the spiritual needs inventory for patients near the end of life. *Oncology Nursing Forum, 33*(4), 737–744.

Jaarsma, T. A., Pool, G., Sanderman, R., & Ranchor, A. V. (2006). Psychometric properties of the Dutch version of the posttraumatic growth inventory among cancer patients. *Psycho-Oncology, 15*(10), 911–920.

Jim, H. S., Purnell, J. Q., Richardson, S. A., Golden-Kreutz, D., & Andersen, B. L. (2006). Measuring meaning in life following cancer. *Quality of Life Research, 15*(8), 1355–1371.

Ka'opua, L. S., Gotay, C. C., & Boehm, P. S. (2007). Spiritually based resources in adaptation to long-term prostate cancer survival: Perspectives of elderly wives. *Health & Social Work, 32*(1), 29–39.

Katerndahl, D. (2008). Impact of spiritual symptoms and their interactions on health services and life satisfaction. *Annals of Family Medicine, 6*(5), 412–420.

Kub, J. E., Nolan, M. T., Hughes, M. T., Terry, P. B., Sulmasy, D. P., Astrow, A., et al., (2003). Religious importance and practices of patients with a life-threatening illness: implications for screening protocols. *Applied Nursing Research, 16*(3), 196–200.

Leak, A., Hu, J., & King, C. R. (2008). Symptom distress, spirituality, and quality of life in African American breast cancer survivors. *Cancer Nursing, 31*(1), E15–21.

McClung, E., Grossoehme, D. H., & Jacobson, A. F. (2006). Collaborating with chaplains to meet spiritual needs. *MEDSURG Nursing, 15*(3), 147–156.

McEwen, M. (2005). Spiritual nursing care: state of the art. *Holistic Nursing Practice, 19*(4), 161–168.

McGrath, P. (2004). Positive outcomes for survivors of haematological malignancies from a spiritual perspective. *International Journal of Nursing Practice, 10*(6), 280–291.

Miller, B. (2005). Spiritual journey during and after cancer treatment. *Gynecologic Oncology, 99,* S129–S130.

Park C. L., & Folkman S. (1997). Meaning in the context of stress and coping. *Rev Gen Psychol, 1*, 115–144.

Peterman, A., Fitchett, G., Brady, M., Hernandez, L., & Cella, D. (2002). Measuring spiritual well-being in people with cancer: The functional assessment of chronic illness therapy-spiritual well-being scale (FACIT-Sp). *Annals of Behavioral Medicine, 24*(1), 49–58.

Puchalski, C., & Romer, A. L. (2000). Taking a spiritual history allows clinicians to understand patients more fully. *Journal of Palliative Medicine, 3*(1), 129–138.

Ramondetta, L. M., & Sills, D. (2004). Spirituality in gynecological oncology: A review. *International Journal of Gynecological Cancer, (14),* 183–201.

Rancour, P. (2008). Using archetypes and transitions theory to help move from active treatment to survivorship. *Clinical Journal of Oncology Nursing, 12*(6), 935–940.

Rumbold, B. (2003). Caring for the Spirit: Lessons from working with the dying. *Medical Journal of Australia, 179,* S11–S13.

Skalla, K., & McCoy, J. (2006). Spiritual assessment of patients with cancer: The moral authority, vocation, aesthetic, social, and transcendent model. *Oncology Nursing Forum, 33*(4), 745–751.

Sulmasy, D. P. (2006). Spiritual issue in the care of dying patients. *Journal of the American Medical Association, 296*(11), 1385–1392.

Tedeschi, R. G., & Calhoun, L. G. (1996). The Posttraumatic Growth Inventory: Measuring the positive legacy of trauma. *Journal of Traumatic Stress, 9*(3), 455–471.

Vachon, M. (2008). Meaning, spirituality, and wellness in cancer survivors. *Seminars in Oncology Nursing, 24*(3), 218–225.

Walter, T. (2002). Spirituality in palliative care: Opportunity or burden? *Palliative Medicine, 16*(2), 133–139.

CHAPTER NINE

Coordination of Care

Charlotte Bell and Lisa Kennedy Sheldon

Oncology nurses, as part of the healthcare team, are in a unique position to help patients navigate, coordinate, and advocate for appropriate care during survivorship. Cancer requires patients to negotiate new relationships with insurers, employers, and even government agencies, especially as they move into survivorship.

Oncology nurses and social workers, as part of the oncology team, are frequently involved in helping patients and their families negotiate the complex policies regarding workplace issues and reimbursement for healthcare services. Additionally, the coordination of care between oncology and primary care providers may become fragmented and incomplete, making it difficult for patients to understand their future care. This section reviews types of healthcare insurance, legislative protection for survivors and persons with disabilities, rights in the workplace, medical leave for patients and their families, disability, and coordination of care among healthcare providers.

Healthcare insurance was originally developed to cover medical expenses. In the United States, health insurance can be provided by private insurers or the government. According to the statistics on health insurance in 2007 from the United States Census Bureau, 67.5% of people had private insurance, 27.8% had government health insurance, and 15.3 % were uninsured. Employers most frequently purchase private insurance for a group of employees.

Government health insurance programs include Medicare and Medicaid, with many people being eligible for dual coverage. General coverage for these programs includes:

- Medicare, a federal program, covers people (and their spouses) aged 65 and over who have paid taxes for 40 or more quarters, and other people who meet special criteria. Medicare has four components of coverage—Part A: Hospital Insurance, Part B: Medical Insurance, Part C: Medicare + Choice and Medicare Advantage to add prescription drug coverage, and Part D: People with Medicare Part or B who purchase a stand-alone Prescription Drug Plan (PDP). Most people with Medicare still have to pay out-of-pocket for copayments, deductibles, and PDP.
- Medicaid, a joint federal and state program, pays for healthcare services for people and families with low incomes and resources, including children, senior citizens, and those with disabilities. It is a needs-based program and has set criteria for poverty, disability, and resources, including homes.

Increasingly, people with any type of healthcare insurance are required to make copayments, deductibles, and/or out-of-pocket expenses before insurance coverage begins to cover the medical care. Coinsurance, a secondary policy, may be purchased to pay for those expenses that the primary insurance does not cover, including prescription medication. Health plans or Health Maintenance Organizations (HMOs) pay a fixed amount of prepaid services; these are frequently called subscription-based health plans.

Negotiating the system to pay for cancer care services is not often simple. Cancer survivors and their families have to deal with deductibles, copayments, exclusions, preauthorization, coverage limits, and network providers. Additionally, they may be unable to work to pay for their premiums and other expenses if the rigors of treatment or the effects of the disease process change their ability to function in the work setting. For patients who become disabled and unable to work, certain protections have been mandated by the government. The Consolidated Omnibus Budget Reconciliation Act of 1985 (COBRA) protects people who can no longer work (a "qualifying event") from loss of insurance coverage by mandating continued healthcare insurance coverage after leaving employment for 18 to 36 months, depending on the event.

Oncology nurses often hear the concerns of survivors and refer them to oncology social workers for help navigating the system. According to the Association of Oncology Social Work (AOSW), oncology social workers are specially trained in cancer care and the goals of clinical practice include the following:

- Fostering coping and adaptation to cancer and its effects in order to help cancer survivors maintain or improve quality of life
- Assisting survivors in navigating healthcare systems to help them achieve quality care
- Mobilizing new or existing family, system, and community resources to provide social and emotional support to cancer survivors
- Conducting research to advance clinical knowledge or evaluate practice effectiveness
- Advocating with, or on behalf of, survivors, families, and caregivers to address their needs, or for policies and programs that will benefit them

As part of the oncology team, social workers can help survivors and their families adapt to a diagnosis of cancer. They also can assist them to navigate the available resources. Some of the most difficult scenarios involve families depleting their resources for medical expenses and no longer able to pay their mortgage, bills, and/or healthcare insurance. Sometimes the money for copayments comes from the food budget for the family. For many people, it is difficult to ask for help and even more humbling to ask for welfare assistance. Oncology social workers are adept at supporting patients and their families, and can offer counseling about financial matters in ways that are sensitive to the concerns and respectful to the individual. They may find sources of support and assistance through state agencies and community groups. Oncology social workers work with oncology nurses, oncologists, and others to help patients afford the care they need.

Supporting families during health crises is one part of oncology care. The Family and Medical Leave Act (FMLA), passed in 1993, allows family members to take up to 12 weeks of unpaid, job-protected leave of absence from their employment to care for a family member or for themselves if they become ill and can no longer work. They may return to their same position or one of equal pay, benefits, and responsibility after the leave. The leave enables both patients and family members to take protected time to care for themselves or each other. Certain paperwork is required from employers that may be completed by an advanced practice nurse or physician.

People with a diagnosis of cancer, even in the distant past, often face various forms of discrimination. Not always obvious, discrimination can occur at the place of employment, from insurance agencies, and even from members in the community.

A cancer diagnosis sometimes creates fear in others, fear about risk, longevity, or impairment. For example, a person who has lost his or her hair from chemotherapy and/or radiation therapy is often viewed differently. The 1990 Americans with Disabilities Act (ADA) falls under the Federal Equal Opportunity (FEO) laws. Job discrimination for cancer patients falls under Title I and V of the ADA, which prohibit employment discrimination against qualified individuals with disabilities in the private sector and state and local governments. Some states have specific laws prohibiting cancer-based discrimination. Private employers and government agencies may not discriminate against qualified people in any of the terms, conditions, and privileges of employment and requires employers to "make reasonable accommodations for people with a disability." People with cancer may require modifications to their work schedule, environment, and travel because of the side effects of the disease and/or treatment. Many people with cancer continue working, but require modifications to be able to continue in their current job. Support from the oncology team may provide the resources and information that people need to continue their roles in the workplace and society.

The Lance Armstrong Foundation recommends specific records that cancer survivors should keep (see Web site in references). These include employment benefits, insurance policies, Medical Information Bureau (MIB) Group Report, Social Security Personal Earnings and Benefit Record, health record, personal finance records, advance directives, and will. The MIB Group Report is the information about a person's medical history that is shared among 500 insurers. Cancer survivors should check the report for accuracy to prevent discrimination.

Cancer survivors often struggle with coordinating their care among multiple healthcare providers. They may have a primary care provider, an oncologist, a radiation oncologist, and a surgeon who have participated in their care. Primary care providers are often concerned about providing careful surveillance for a cancer diagnosis and defer to the oncology specialists. Survivors can advocate for their care during follow-up by asking who they should see, what tests should be scheduled, and who will be coordinating their care. It is often best for survivors to continue to see their primary care provider for all routine health screenings and problems and also create a follow-up schedule with their cancer care providers. They can recommend that each provider sends the other providers copies of visits with recommendations for follow-up visits and testing. Most importantly, cancer survivors should find a primary provider they feel comfortable talking with as they move into the future (Feuerstein & Findley, 2006).

A treatment summary is a useful tool for survivors and healthcare providers. It condenses and summarizes the cancer treatment and follow-up and surveillance. Increasingly, providers are using a treatment summary to help coordinate care among providers and empower the survivor with information about the often complex care they received to treat the cancer. The American Society of Clinical Oncology (ASCO) has completed a general treatment summary as well as templates for two specific cancers, breast cancer and colorectal cancer, with more templates in development. Treatment summaries are useful to survivors and healthcare providers as well as in the ongoing monitoring of quality of cancer care (Ganz, 2007). The treatment summary may consist of three parts, depending on the patient's cancer and treatment plan:

- A summary of surgical treatment particularly the operative report and pathology
- A summary of radiation treatment, including the reason for irradiation, the area, and the dose delivered
- A summary of the chemotherapy regimen, specifically the drugs administered, how the patient tolerated the treatment, including toxicities, and the outcomes of care

The treatment summary also should indicate the patient's response to treatment(s), including tumor markers and evidence from radiologic tests, treatment for side effects and toxicities such as hospitalizations and additional treatment, and potential late effects of treatment. Additionally, the summary should address psychosocial needs and concerns and long-term plan of care, specific providers and their responsibilities in follow-up care, results of genetic testing, and recommendations for healthy behaviors.

The Lance Armstrong Foundation also provides specific guidelines for organizing medical records. At a minimum, a treatment summary should include:

- Date of diagnosis
- Type of cancer
- Pathology report with staging
- Places and dates of specific treatments, including details of surgery, sites and amounts of radiation therapy, names and doses of chemotherapy, and supportive drugs such as growth factors
- Essential reports, including laboratory testing, x-rays, CAT scans and MRIs
- Problems that occurred during treatment and their management
- Hospitalizations
- Long-term effects of treatment that may occur
- Medications, including supportive drugs such as growth factors, nutritional supplements and vitamins, as well as allergies
- Contact information for all providers involved in the care

A survivorship care plan is another useful tool to help both cancer survivors and healthcare providers communicate and coordinate care. Because cancer survivors may have several healthcare providers participating in their care, survivors often are left to coordinate their care.

Other healthcare providers may include a second opinion at another healthcare institution, clinical trials nurses, social workers, therapists, nutritionists, practitioners providing complementary therapy such as acupuncture, and physical and occupational therapists. It is important to encourage survivors to keep complete records, including contact information for people who have participated in their care.

A survivorship care plan is one method of consolidating the recommendations for future care. It should contain several essential components to ensure adequate surveillance and follow-up after cancer treatment. Surveillance generally consists of office visits and testing, including blood work, endoscopy, surgery, and/or radiologic tests. These tests allow for early detection and treatment of recurrences as well as screening for secondary malignancies.

The oncology team provides a variety of services for people with a cancer diagnosis and facilitates their journey through the healthcare system and into survivorship. Oncology nurses and oncology social workers work with physicians, pastoral care, and other providers to deliver comprehensive and supportive care. Some facets of cancer care can be challenging including working with employers and insurers. Oncology social workers have the background to help survivors navigate the system and locate resources to allow them to remain financially sound during and after cancer treatment. Oncology nurses are ideally suited to coordinate care within the oncology team and with primary care providers, and help survivors locate and maximize available services.

References

Feuerstein, M., & Findley, P. (2006). The Cancer Survivor's Guide: The Essential Handbook to Life after Cancer. New York: Marlowe and Company, Avalon Publishing Group Incorporated.

Ganz, P. A. (2007). Cancer survivorship: Today and tomorrow. New York: Springer Science+Business Media.

Bibliography

Feuerstein, M. (2007). *Handbook of cancer survivorship*. New York: Springer Science+Business Media.

Hewitt, M., Greenfield, S., & Stovall, E. (2005). *From cancer patient to cancer survivor: Lost in transition*. Washington, DC: The National Academies Press.

Institute of Medicine of the National Academies. (2007). *Implementing cancer survivorship planning: Workshop summary*. Washington, DC: The National Academies Press.

Web Sites

Association of Oncology Social Work (AOSW). Retrieved January 20, 2009. http://www.aosw.org/html/prof-scope.php

United States Census Bureau. Health Insurance. Retrieved January 20, 2009. http://www.census.gov/hhes/www/hlthins/lilthin07/hlth07asc.html

Consolidated Omnibus Budget Reconciliation Act of 1985 (COBRA). Accessed January 20, 2009. http://www.cobrainsurance.cc/

Family Medical Leave Act (FMLA) of 1993. Accessed January 20, 2009. http://www.dol.gov/esa/whd/regs/statutes/fmla.htm

1990 Americans with Disabilities Act (ADA). Accessed January 20, 2009. http://www.ada.gov/pubs/ada.htm

The Lance Armstrong Foundation. Important Records Survivors Should Keep. Accessed January 20, 2009. http://www.livestrong.org/site/c.khLXK1PxHmF/b.2662483/k.1C4F/Important_Records_Survivors_Should_Keep.htm\

Working It Out, Your Employment Rights As A Cancer Survivor, Barbara Hoffman, JD, National Coalition for Cancer Survivorship (NCCS), 2008. Accessed January 21, 2009. http://www.canceradvocacy.org/resources/publications/employment.pdf

Federal Laws Prohibiting Job Discrimination Questions and Answers, Federal Equal Employment Opportunity (EEO) Laws. Accessed January 21, 2009. http://www.eeoc.gov/facts/qanda.html

Facing Forward, Life After Cancer Treatment, A Guide for People Who Were Treated for Cancer. U.S. Department of Health and Human Services, National Institute of Health, National Cancer Institute, NCI Publication No. 02-2424, Printed May 2002, pp. 89–93. http://www.cancer.gov/cancertopics/life-after-treatment

Web Sites

Americans with Disabilities Act: Accessed July 14, 2009: http://www.ada.gov/

Cancer Care: Professional care for people affected by cancer. Accessed July 14, 2009: http://www.cancercare.org

Cancer and Careers: A resource for working women with cancer. Accessed November 18, 2008 from www.cancerandcareers.org

Consolidated Omnibus Budget Reconciliation Act (COBRA). Accessed November 16, 2008 from http://www.dol.gov/dol/topic/health plans/cobra.htm

Lance Armstrong Foundation. LIVESTRONG. Accessed November 16, 2008 from www.livestrong.org

Resources

American Cancer Society. (2008). *Cancer facts and figures: 2008*. Atlanta: Author.

Centers for Disease Control and Prevention. *A national action plan for cancer survivorship: Advancing public health policies*. (2004). Atlanta: Author.

Feuerstein, M. (2007). *Handbook of cancer survivorship*. New York. Springer Science+Business Media.

Hewitt, M., Greenfield, S., & Stovall, E. (2005). *From cancer patient to cancer survivor: Lost in transition*. Washington, DC: The National Academies Press.

Institute of Medicine of the National Academies. (2007). *Implementing cancer survivorship planning: Workshop summary*. Washington, DC: The National Academies Press.

Institute of Medicine: National Cancer Policy Forum. (2009, in press). *Ensuring quality cancer care through the oncology workforce: sustaining care in the 21st century: Workshop Summary*. Washington DC. The National Academies Press.

Specific References: Colorectal Cancer

ASCO Patient Guide. (2008). *Follow-up care for colorectal cancer*. Retrieved November 15, 2008 from http://www.cancer.net/patient/ASCO+Resources/What+to+Know:+ASCO's+Guidelines/What+to+Know:+ASCO's+Guideline+on+Follow-Up+Care+for+Colorectal+Cancer

Memorial Sloan-Kettering Cancer Center. (2008). *Prediction tools: Colorectal nomogram*. Retrieved December 2, 2008 from http://www.mskcc.org/mskcc/html/83364.cfm

National Cancer Institute. (2008). *Colon and rectal cancer*. Retrieved December 2, 2008 from http://www.cancer.gov/cancertopics/pdq/treatment/colon/HealthProfessional/